Size and Strength Blueprint

■ ■ ■

The Ultimate Encyclopedia of Proven Workouts

By Josh Bryant
and
Noah Bryant

Size and Strength Blueprint

By Josh Bryant and Noah Bryant

ISBN-13: 9781505832440

Contents

Dedication

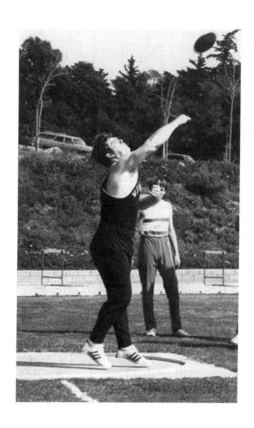

To our father, who has always loved us unconditionally
and believed that we could do anything we put our minds to.
Every parenting decision we make, we look to your example.

Introduction

"There's a young man down the street from me who trains with weights. He's been at it for about three years now but you'd never know to look at him. He's got no build at all. My grandmother has been dead for 12 years and she probably still looks better than he does."

This boy, so poetically described by immortal iron game author John McCallum, is exactly who we do not want you to become. We want you to realize all of your physique and strength goals, reaping the rewards for your hours of hard work in the weight room.

Like our father always says, "The road to hell is paved with good intentions." No matter how well-intentioned your lifting program is, you need a well thought out plan to achieve your goals.

This encyclopedia gives you that plan!

No longer will you have to ask yourself, "What am I going to do in the gym today?" You have in your hands the key to unlock your potential.

Think of this compendium as your blueprint, and of yourself as the hard-nosed, no-nonsense contractor. The blueprint gives you the information you need to build the house (location of walls, ceiling height, door placement, etc.). However, without your nose to the grindstone, the house will never be built.

Without blueprints from the architect, you, the contractor, will go around building the same house repeatedly. You will build the same floor plan, paint the same color, and construct the same ol' boring house, month after month and year after year. My guess is the jobs will dry up and you will have to find a new line of work. You see, we need new blueprints (or workouts) if we want to make progress.

From the most experienced gym rat to the PhD in exercise physiology, it is very challenging to continually create fresh and effective workouts. Folks need something fresh and inspiring, and also something that is effective and produces results — not some circus sideshow workout. The plans in this book hit that sweet spot.

You now have access to 12-week periodized training plans and fresh ideas for single bodybuilding workouts.

The ideas and plans presented in this book have been tested on top-ranked IFBB pro bodybuilders, a multitude of world record setting strength athletes, and middle-aged men and women with full time jobs and families.

First and foremost we are trainers, not writers talking about theoretical workout plans. These workouts have been tested and proven on ourselves and our clients.

Whenever you need something new and effective for yourself or your personal training clients, come back to your blueprint.

Remember, the journey of 10,000 miles starts with the first step. You have taken the first step by purchasing the blueprint; now you must read and continue your strength journey.

Strength and health are a lifestyle. Thank you for letting us be a part of your lifestyle and journey.

WHOLE BODY WORKOUTS

■ ■ ■
Size & Strength Stampede:
The Flagship 12 Week Program

This 12 week cycle consists of 3 distinct phases. These three phases, put together, will open the gates to an anabolic Valhalla and build Herculean levels of strength to match.

During the first three weeks you will more than likely feel beaten and broken down. And just when you

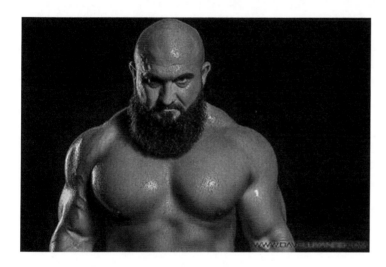

think you can't take anymore, your body will start to adapt to the barbaric amounts of volume, giving you the foundation needed to plow through and maximize the subsequent two phases.

Beginning with the first workout, you're training with the right combo of compound movements, isolation movements and volume to catalyze results immediately.

For most readers, we are training at an entirely new level of intensity with the traditional exercises, and throwing in some movements you are not accustomed to that require extreme concentration and coordination.

Just when you think you cannot take any more, Week 4 is a deload. The deload gives your Central Nervous System (CNS), joints, and muscles a well-deserved break and also minimizes the chance of overtraining and the risk of injury.

Many folks grow on the deload because after three weeks of "tearing down," a deload offers the opportunity to "build up."

The primary objective of Phase 1 is to build a base!

Phase 1
Here are some guidelines to follow:

- Follow each workout in the recommended sequence, religiously adhering to the rest intervals.
- Sometimes the same exercise may be repeated twice—that is not a typo, but rather a foundational movement you will perform in a different way. The first way is the most important way, that's why we are hitting it when you are fresh.

- When performing the unilateral exercises (one limb at a time), ALWAYS START WITH THE WEAKER SIDE, simply because your energy levels are fresh. Our goal is for structural balance, and it will not be a problem to match reps on the weaker side.
- Consecutive exercises with an A & B pairing mean they can be performed consecutively in a superset fashion, immediately moving from exercise A to B. The rest interval is between supersets.
- If weights are not listed, go as heavy as possible without sacrificing form.
- On max-reps sets do as many as possible, stopping one shy of failure or technical breakdown.

All percentages are based off of a one-rep max of prescribed lift unless otherwise noted. Make sure you start with accurate one-rep maxes; advanced lifters need to base the listed percentages in the program with 95 percent of their one-rep max.

Phase 1 - Volume Phase
Week 1

Day 1	Rest Interval	REPS	SETS	Day 2	Rest Interval	REPS	SETS
Bench Press 75% set 1, 80% set 2	As needed	3	2	Squat 75% (last set as many reps as possible)	As needed	5	5
Bench Press sets 65% (last set as many reps as possible)	60 seconds	6	4	Front Squat 70% of back squat, used for exercise 1	60 seconds	2	6
Incline Press (A)	90 seconds	6	4	Walking 45-Degree Plate Lunge	60 seconds	20 yards	2
Chin-Up (B)		5 (if you can do more, add weight)	5	Single Leg Curl (A)	60 seconds	6	3
Incline Fly (A)	90 second	12	3	Leg Extension (B)		30	3
Single-Arm Eccentric Barbell Curl (B)	90 seconds	3	3	Single-Leg Glute Bridge (A)	30 seconds	12	3
Incline Dumbbell Curl (A)	60 seconds	8,12,15	3	Mini-Band Clamshell (B)		10	3
Incline I-Y-T (B)	60 seconds	10 reps each/30 reps total	3	Front Squat Static Hold 15 sec (Back Squat Weight Exercise 1)	45 seconds	1	2
Side Plank	45 seconds	20 seconds	2	Calf Raise Standing	45 seconds	15	3
Day 3	**Rest Interval**	**REPS**	**SETS**	**Day 4**	**Rest Interval**	**REPS**	**SETS**
Standing Overhead Press (75 %) Last Set Max Reps	45 seconds	2	8	Squats (65%)	30 sec	1	6
Crucifix Hold (Hold 30 Seconds)		30 seconds	1	Deadlift (77.5%)		3	1
Rear Delt Fly (A)	45 seconds	12	3	Deadlift (all sets 65%)	60 seconds	4	6
Lateral Raise on Incline with 5 second Eccentric (B)	60 seconds	5	3	Dumbbell Shrug	60 seconds	12	3
Dicks Press	90 seconds	12	4	Pendlay Row	60 seconds	5	4
Weighted Dips (A)	120 seconds	6	3	Dumbbell Pullover (A)	75 seconds	12	3
Overhead Rope Ext (B)	45 seconds	15	3	Straight Arm Pulldown (B)	45 seconds	12	4
				Weighted Neutral Grip Pull-up	45 seconds	3	6
				Sledgehammer (maximum reps each way for 30 seconds)	75 seconds	Maximum	3
				Sled Drags Optional)	60 seconds	20 yards	6
				Spread V Leg Raise	45 seconds	6	3

Phase 1 - Volume Phase

Week 2

Day 1	Rest Interval	REPS	SETS	Day 2	Rest Interval	REPS	SETS
Bench Press 77% set 1, 83% set 2	As needed	3	2	Squat 80% (last set as many reps as possible)	As needed	5	5
Bench Press sets 65% (last set as many reps as possible)	60 seconds	7	4	Front Squat 70% of back squat, used for exercise 1	60 seconds	2	6
Incline Press (A)	90 seconds	6	4	Walking 45-Degree Plate Lunge	60 seconds	20 yards	2
Chin-Up (B)		5 (if you can do more, add weight)	5	Single Leg Curl (A)	60 seconds	7	3
Incline Fly (A)	90 second	15	3	Leg Extension (B)		25	3
Single-Arm Eccentric Barbell Curl (B)	90 seconds	4	3	Single-Leg Glute Bridge (A)	30 seconds	12	3
Incline Dumbbell Curl (A)	60 seconds	6,10,12	3	Mini-Band Clamshell (B)		10	3
Incline I-Y-T (B)	60 seconds	10 reps each/30 reps total	3	Front Squat Static Hold 15 sec (Back Squat Weight Exercise 1)	45 seconds	1	2
Side Plank	45 seconds	20 seconds	2	Calf Raise Standing	45 seconds	13	3
Day 3	Rest Interval	REPS	SETS	Day 4	Rest Interval	REPS	SETS
Standing Overhead Press (77.5 %) Last Set Max Reps	45 seconds	2	8	Squats (65%)	30 sec	1	6
Crucifix Hold (Hold 35 Seconds)		35 seconds	1	Deadlift (82%)		3	1
Rear Delt Fly (A)	45 seconds	13	3	Deadlift (all sets 65%)	60 seconds	4	8
Lateral Raise on Incline with 5 second Eccentric (B)	60 seconds	6	3	Dumbbell Shrug	60 seconds	15	3
Dicks Press	90 seconds	10	4	Pendlay Row	60 seconds	5	5
Weighted Dips (A)	120 seconds	5	3	Dumbbell Pullover (A)	75 seconds	13	3
Overhead Rope Ext (B)	45 seconds	15	3	Straight Arm Pulldown (B)	45 seconds	15	4
				Weighted Neutral Grip Pull-up	45 seconds	4	6
				Sledgehammer (maximum reps each way for 35 seconds)	75 seconds	Maximum	3
				Sled Drags (Optional)	60 seconds	20 yards	6
				Spread V Leg Raise	45 seconds	6	3

Phase 1 - Volume Phase							
Week 3							
Day 1	Rest Interval	REPS	SETS	Day 2	Rest Interval	REPS	SETS
Bench Press 79% set 1, 86% set 2	As needed	3	2	Squat 83% (last set as many reps as possible)	As needed	5	5
Bench Press sets 65% (last set as many reps as possible)	60 seconds	5	8	Front Squat 70% of back squat, used for exercise 1	60 seconds	2	6
Incline Press (A)	90 seconds	5	4	Walking 45-Degree Plate Lunge	60 seconds	20 yards	2
Chin-Up (B)		5 (if you can do more, add weight)	5	Single Leg Curl (A)	60 seconds	8	3
Incline Fly (A)	90 second	15	3	Leg Extension (B)		20	3
Single-Arm Eccentric Barbell Curl (B)	90 seconds	5	3	Single-Leg Glute Bridge (A)	30 seconds	12	3
Incline Dumbbell Curl (A)	60 seconds	5,8,12	3	Mini-Band Clamshell (B)		10	3
Incline I-Y-T (B)	60 seconds	10 reps each/30 reps total	3	Front Squat Static Hold 15 sec (Back Squat Weight Exercise 1)	45 seconds	1	2
Side Plank	45 seconds	20 seconds	2	Calf Raise Standing	45 seconds	12	3
Day 3	Rest Interval	REPS	SETS	Day 4	Rest Interval	REPS	SETS
Standing Overhead Press (80%) Last Set Max Reps	45 seconds	2	8	Squats (65%)	30 sec	1	6
Crucifix Hold (Hold 40 Seconds)		40 seconds	1	Deadlift (86%)		3	1
Rear Delt Fly (A)	45 seconds	13	3	Deadlift (all sets 65%)	60 seconds	4	10
Lateral Raise on Incline with 5 second Eccentric (B)	60 seconds	6	3	Dumbbell Shrug	60 seconds	10	3
Dicks Press	90 seconds	8	4	Pendlay Row	60 seconds	5	5
Weighted Dips (A)	120 seconds	5	3	Dumbbell Pullover (A)	75 seconds	15	3
Overhead Rope Ext (B)	45 seconds	15	3	Straight Arm Pulldown (B)	45 seconds	15	4
				Weighted Neutral Grip Pull-up	45 seconds	3	6
				Sledgehammer (maximum reps each way for 40 seconds)	75 seconds	Maximum	3
				Sled Drags (Optional)	60 seconds	20 yards	6
				Spread V Leg Raise	45 seconds	6	3

Week 4 is a deload—use 70 percent of the weight used for each exercise and do 70 percent of the sets; so three sets would be (3 x .7=2.1). Round to the nearest whole number. On the deload, three sets would become two sets and 200 pounds would become 140 pounds.

Phase 2

You made it past the toughest stage — congratulations! You are now entering Phase 2, or the "Piecing it Together Phase."

You should look and feel better, because you are obviously a lot stronger. Instead of becoming complacent, let's kick it into high gear and go to that next level.

We are going to add in some partial movements to overload your muscles with the purpose of elevating strength potential when performing the same exercises with their full range of motion. We are also going to increase the intensity.

No access to boards? No worries, you can also use a piece of Styrofoam that is roughly the same size. EliteFTS sells a great device called the "Shoulder Saver" that many lifters prefer to boards.

If you don't have an ab wheel do not worry, as one can be purchased for as little as five bucks online. Getting ahold of a large tractor tire is easy and inexpensive because it costs the businesses that handle used tires a lot of money to dispose of them, so expect them to beg you to take them off their hands! Unless you live in Outer Mongolia, a quick Google search will yield scores of spots to grab a tire.

Phase 2 - Piecing It Together Phase
Week 5

Day 1	Rest Interval	REPS	SETS	Day 2	Rest Interval	REPS	SETS
Bench Press 83% set 1, 88% set 2	As needed	3	2	Squat 82%, 87%	As needed	4	2
Bench Press sets 75% (last set as many reps as possible)	90 seconds	5	4	Squat 75% (last set as many reps as possible)	75 sec	4	4
3 Board Press (Set 1 85%, set 2 90%, Set 3 95%)	150 sec	5,4,3	3	Zercher Squat 70% of back squat, used for exercise 1	90 seconds	3	4
Dead Bench Press (1.5 inches off Chest), Max out to Establish 1 RM	180 seconds	1	3	Tire Flip	60 seconds	5	3
Scapular Retraction (A)	45 sec	12	3	Glute Ham Raise	60 seconds	6	3
Incline Cable Fly (B)		15	3	Single Leg Press (A)	75 sec	12	3
Chin-up (A) Add as much weight as possible	120 seconds	5	3	Single-Leg Glute Bridge (B)		12	3
Zottman Curls (B)		12,10,8	3	Front Squat Static Hold 15 sec (Back Squat Weight Exercise 1)	45 seconds	1	2
Side Plank	45 seconds	20 seconds	2	Calf Raise Standing	45 seconds	12	3
Day 3	**Rest Interval**	**REPS**	**SETS**	**Day 4**	**Rest Interval**	**REPS**	**SETS**
Standing Overhead Press (all sets 83%) Last Set as Many Reps as possible	90 sec	2	6	Squats (65%)	30 sec	1	6
Seated Military Press (overload) 3 inch Range of Motion In Squat Rack off pins, as heavy as possible	As needed	5	3	Deadlift (90%)		2	1
Shoulder Box	60 seconds	12	3	Deadlift (all sets 73%)	75 seconds	3	6
Flat Bench Reverse Fly (A)	45 seconds	12	3	Trap Bar Shrug	90 seconds	12	3
Cable Lateral Raise (B)		12	3	T-bar Prison Rows	90 seconds	6	4
Close-Grip Decline Press (75% of Bench Press 1 RM) Second Set as many reps as possible	180 seconds	6	2	Dumbbell Pullover (A)	75 seconds	15	3
Rolling Dumbbell Triceps Ext	45 seconds	15	3	Farmers Walk (B)	90 seconds	20 yds	2
				Weighted Neutral Grip Pull ups (A)	150 seconds	3	4
				Side Medicine Ball Toss (B)	90 seconds	4	4

	Phase 2 - Piecing It Together Phase						
			Week 6				
Day 1	Rest Interval	REPS	SETS	Day 2	Rest Interval	REPS	SETS
Bench Press 85% set 1, 91% set 2	As needed	3	2	Squat 92%		3	1
Bench Press sets 77.5% (last set as many reps as possible)	90 seconds	4	5	Squat 80% (last set as many reps as possible)	90 sec	4	4
3 Board Press (Set 1 85%, set 2 95%, Set 3 100%)	150 sec	5,3,1	3	Zercher Squat 70% of back squat, used for exercise 1	90 seconds	3	4
Dead Bench Press (1.5 inches off Chest) 80%	60 seconds	1	6	Tire Flip	60 seconds	6	3
Scapular Retraction (A)	45 sec	12	3	Glute Ham Raise	60 seconds	6	3
Incline Cable Fly (B)		15	3	Single Leg Press (A)	75 sec	12	3
Chin-up (A) Add as much weight as possible	120 seconds	4	3	Single-Leg Glute Bridge (B)		12	3
Zottman Curls (B)		10,9,8	3	Front Squat Static Hold 15 sec (Back Squat Weight Exercise 1)	45 seconds	1	2
Side Plank	45 seconds	20 seconds	2	Calf Raise Standing	45 seconds	12	3
Day 3	Rest Interval	REPS	SETS	Day 4	Rest Interval	REPS	SETS
Standing Overhead Press (all sets 85%) Last Set as Many Reps as possible	90 sec	2	6	Squats (65%)	30 sec	1	6
Seated Military Press (overload) 3 inch Range of Motion in Squat Rack off pins, as heavy as possible	As needed	5,4,3	3	Deadlift (95%)		2	1
Shoulder Box	60 seconds	12	3	Deadlift (all sets 77%)	75 seconds	3	5
Flat Bench Reverse Fly (A)	45 seconds	14	3	Trap Bar Shrug	90 seconds	12	3
Cable Lateral Raise (B)		15	3	T-bar Prison Rows	90 seconds	6	4
Close-Grip Decline Press (78% of Bench Press 1 RM) Second Set as many reps as possible	180 seconds	5	2	Dumbbell Pullover (A)	75 seconds	15	3
Rolling Dumbbell Triceps Ext	45 seconds	15	3	Farmers Walk (B)	90 seconds	20 yds	2
				Weighted Neutral Grip Pull ups (A)	150 seconds	3	4
				Side Medicine Ball Toss (B)	90 seconds	4	4

Phase 2 - Piecing It Together Phase							
			Week 7				
Day 1	Rest Interval	REPS	SETS	Day 2	Rest Interval	REPS	SETS
Bench Press 97%		2	1	Squat 98%		2	1
Bench Press sets 80% (last set as many reps as possible)	90 seconds	3	5	Squat 83% (last set as many reps as possible)	90 sec	3	4
3 Board 95%, 102%, 107%	150 sec	1	3	Zercher Squat 70% of back squat, used for exercise 1	90 seconds	3	4
Dead Bench Press (1.5 Inches off Chest) 85%	60 seconds	1	5	Tire Flip	60 seconds	6	3
Scapular Retraction (A)	45 sec	12	3	Glute Ham Raise	60 seconds	6	3
Incline Cable Fly (B)		15	3	Single Leg Press (A)	75 sec	12	3
Chin-up (A) Add as much weight as possible	120 seconds	3	3	Single-Leg Glute Bridge (B)		12	3
Zottman Curls (B)		10,8,6	3	Front Squat Static Hold 15 sec (Back Squat Weight Exercise 1)	45 seconds	1	2
Side Plank	45 seconds	20 seconds	2	Calf Raise Standing	45 seconds	12	3
Day 3	Rest Interval	REPS	SETS	Day 4	Rest Interval	REPS	SETS
Standing Overhead Press (all sets 88%) Last Set as Many Reps as possible	90 sec	3,2,1,3,2,1	6	Squats (65%)	30 sec	1	6
Seated Military Press (overload) 3 inch Range of Motion In Squat Rack off pins, as heavy as possible	As needed	3,2,1	3	Deadlift (100%)		2	1
Shoulder Box	60 seconds	12	3	Deadlift (all sets 80%)	75 seconds	3	5
Flat Bench Reverse Fly (A)	45 seconds	14	3	Trap Bar Shrug	90 seconds	12	3
Cable Lateral Raise (B)		15	3	T-bar Prison Rows	90 seconds	5	4
Close-Grip Decline Press (80% of Bench Press 1 RM) Second Set as many reps as possible	180 seconds	5	2	Dumbbell Pullover (A)	75 seconds	15	3
Rolling Dumbbell Triceps Ext	45 seconds	15	3	Farmers Walk (B)	90 seconds	20 yds	2
				Weighted Neutral Grip Pull ups (A)	150 seconds	4	4
				Side Medicine Ball Toss (B)	90 seconds	4	4

Week 8 is another deload week. Follow directions for Week 4.

Phase 3

You've gotta be loving the gains by now!

Just when things seem too good to be true, the final icing will be put on the cake, concluding in a more muscular, functional, and stronger you.

How can we do this? By taking intensity to a new level, the groundwork has been laid with your weeks of high-volume, foundational work.

During the next four weeks, the amount of sets you'll perform on the primary exercises will decrease, while the rest intervals between each set will increase. This will allow your body more time to recover, permitting you to reach new maximum strength totals in each of the core lift exercises.

To handle even heavier weights, the Three-Board Press will become a Five-Board Press; because of this decreased range of motion, we have one objective... HEAVY!

Phase 3 - Reap the Rewards Phase
Week 9

Day 1	Rest Interval	REPS	SETS	Day 2	Rest Interval	REPS	SETS
Bench Press 102%		1	1	Squat 106%		1	1
Bench Press sets 83% (last set as many reps as possible)	90 seconds	2	5	Squat Walkout hold 5 sec do not squat 115%		1	1
Five-Board Press (set 1 90%, set 2 100%, set 3 108%)	150 sec	6,4,3	3	Squat (all sets 86%)	120 seconds	2	4
Paused Bench Press (hold 1 inch off chest for 3 seconds) 65%,70%,75%	180 seconds	3	3	Olympic Pause Squat	120 seconds	3	2
Scapular Retraction (A)	45 sec	12	3	Single-Leg Romanian Deadlift	60 seconds	3	3
Neutral Grip Pull-ups (B) Add as much weight as possible	120 seconds	5	3	Calf Raise Standing	45 seconds	15	3
Gironda Perfect Curls	75 sec	10,8,6	3	Standing Cable Crunch	45 seconds	12	3
Side Plank	45 seconds	20 seconds	2				
Day 3	**Rest Interval**	**REPS**	**SETS**	**Day 4**	**Rest Interval**	**REPS**	**SETS**
Standing Overhead Press (all sets 92%) last set max reps	90 sec	1	4	Squats	30 seconds	1	6
Flat Bench Reverse Fly (A)	45 seconds	15	3	Deadlift 106%	As needed	1	1
Close Grip Bench Press 80% of 1 RM BENCH PRESS (B) Last Set Max Reps	120 seconds	3	3	Deadlift 80%	90 seconds	2	6
Pull over to Press (Close-Grip w/ ez curl bar)	90 seconds	12	3	One Arm Barbell Shrug Smith Machine	90 seconds	12	3
Dumbbell Pause Floor Extension	45 seconds	15	3	One Arm Dumbbell Row	90 seconds	6	4
				Land Mine	45 seconds	8	3

Phase 3 - Reap the Rewards Phase
Week 10

Day 1	Rest Interval	REPS	SETS	Day 2	Rest Interval	REPS	SETS
Bench Press 105%		1	1	Squat 111%		1	1
Bench Press sets 85% (last set as many reps as possible)	90 seconds	2	3	Squat Walkout hold 5 sec do not squat 120%		1	1
Five-Board Press (set 1 90%, set 2 105%, set 3 115%)	150 sec	5,3,1	3	Squat (all sets 88%)	120 seconds	2	3
Paused Bench Press (hold 1 inch off chest for 3 seconds) 65%,73%,79%	180 seconds	3	3	Olympic Pause Squat	120 seconds	3	2
Scapular Retraction (A)	45 sec	12	3	Single-Leg Romanian Deadlift	60 seconds	3	3
Neutral Grip Pull-ups (B) Add as much weight as possible	120 seconds	4	3	Calf Raise Standing	45 seconds	15	3
Gironda Perfect Curls	75 sec	10,8,6	3	Standing Cable Crunch	45 seconds	12	3
Side Plank	45 seconds	20 seconds	2				
Day 3	**Rest Interval**	**REPS**	**SETS**	**Day 4**	**Rest Interval**	**REPS**	**SETS**
Standing Overhead Press (all sets 94%) last set max reps	120 sec	1	3	Squats	30 seconds	1	6
Flat Bench Reverse Fly (A)	45 seconds	15	3	Deadlift 111%		1	1
Grip Bench Press 82% of 1 RM BENCH PRESS (B) Last Set Max Reps	120 seconds	3	3	Deadlift 83%	90 seconds	2	4
Pull over to Press (Close-Grip w/ ez curl bar)	90 seconds	12	3	One Arm Barbell Shrug Smith Machine	90 seconds	10	3
Dumbbell Pause Floor Extension	45 seconds	12	3	One Arm Dumbbell Row	90 seconds	6	4
				Land Mine	45 seconds	8	3

Phase 3 - Reap the Rewards Phase							
Week 11							
Day 1	Rest Interval	REPS	SETS	Day 2	Rest Interval	REPS	SETS
Bench Press 108%		1	1	Squat 114%		1	1
Bench Press sets 87% (last set as many reps as possible)	90 seconds	2	3	Single-Leg Romanian Deadlift	60 seconds	3	3
Five-Board Press Max out	150 sec	1	3	Calf Raise Standing	45 seconds	15	3
Paused Bench Press (hold 1 inch off chest for 3 seconds) 65%,76%,82%	180 seconds	2	3	Standing Cable Crunch	45 seconds	12	3
Scapular Retraction (A)	45 sec	12	3				
Neutral Grip Pull-ups (B) Add as much weight as possible	120 seconds	4	3				
Gironda Perfect Curls	75 sec	10,8,6	3				
Side Plank	45 seconds	20 seconds	2				
Day 3	Rest Interval	REPS	SETS	Day 4	Rest Interval	REPS	SETS
Standing Overhead Press 85%,95%,105%	120 sec	1	3	Squats	30 seconds	1	6
Flat Bench Reverse Fly (A)	45 seconds	15	3	Deadlift 114		1	1
Grip Bench Press 84% of 1 RM BENCH PRESS (B) Last Set Max Reps	120 seconds	3	3	One Arm Barbell Shrug Smith Machine	90 seconds	10	3
Pull over to Press (Close-Grip w/ez curl bar)	90 seconds	12	3	One Arm Dumbbell Row	90 seconds	6	4
Dumbbell Pause Floor Extension	45 seconds	10	3	Land Mine	45 seconds	8	3

Week 12 is a deload week, follow the same prescription as Weeks 4 and 8.

Final Thoughts

Your strength and size are now to a whole new level!

If Week 11 lifts did not satisfy you, don't worry. After deloading during week 12, test your maxes again during week 13.

Your mind, body and spirit are now stronger — congratulations; this program is not for the faint of heart!

I do not recommend running this cycle more than twice a year.

Good luck and good gains!

Time to hit the pig iron!

8 Week Strength-Maximizing Program

Bigger Faster Stronger (BFS) is the name of a popular mass-market strength and conditioning program for high school athletics. The premise is that all athletes want to get bigger, faster and stronger.

Universally, ALL athletes do want to get faster and stronger, but bigger is not always better. As my mentor, Dr. Fred Hatfield, says, "In all the world of sports, speed is king!" The base for speed and athletics is strength. To maximize speed, an athlete should strive for a 2.5-times bodyweight deadlift.

For some NFL linemen, this would be well over 700 pounds. Until you reach this suggested landmark, you will automatically get faster by increasing your strength, assuming bodyweight doesn't balloon up with strength increases.

The truth is, not everyone wants to get bigger.

MMA, boxing, wrestling, powerlifting and a host of other sports require athletes to stay within the parameters of a weight class. Maximizing strength-to-bodyweight ratio is paramount to success in any sport broken into weight classes.

In sprinting, one of the key variables in the speed quotient is strength-to-bodyweight ratio. Of course, it is essential to keep body fat to a minimum, BUT even non-functional, pumped-up muscle mass will slow down a sprinter.

We are not training for the pump with this program—we are training the skill of strength!

Want to maximize muscles mass? GREAT... do another program. Want to maximize strength and minimize mass gains? This is the program for you!

Day	Exercise	Sets/Reps Week 1	Sets/Reps Week 2	Sets/Reps Week 3	Sets/Reps Week 4/Deload
		8 Week Plan			
		Weeks 1-4			
Day 1	Barbell Squat	6x3 (75%; Rest 60 Sec.)	6x3 (80%; Rest 90 Sec.)	6x3 (85%; Rest 120 Sec.)	3x3 (60%; Rest 60 Sec.)
	Barbell Front Squat	3x3	3x3	3x3	3x3 (70% of weight used on week 3)
	Reverse Hack Squat Good Mornings	3x8	3x7	3x6	3x6 (70% of weight used on week 3)
	Pistol Squats	3x3	3x5	3x7	3x3 (70% of weight used on week 3)
	Glute Ham Raises	3x6	3x6	3x6	3x6 (70% of weight used on week 3)
	Land Mines	3x8	3x8	3x8	2x8 (70% of weight used on week 3)
	Standing Weighted Crunches	3x10	3x12	3x12	2x8 (70% of weight used on week 3)
Day 2	Bench Press	6x3 (75%; Rest 60 Sec.)	6x3 (80%; Rest 75 Sec.)	6x3 (85%; Rest 90 Sec.)	3x3 (60%; Rest 60 Sec.)
	Standing Overhead Press	6x1 (75%; Rest 60 Sec.)	6x1 (80%; Rest 60 Sec.)	6x1 (85%; Rest 60 Sec.)	6x1 (60%; Rest 60 Sec.)
	Dead Bench Press	8x1 (65%; Rest 30 Sec.)	8x1 (70%; Rest 40 Sec.)	7x1 (75%; Rest 50 Sec.)	6x1 (60%; Rest 60 Sec.)
	Dicks Press	3x8	3x8	3x8	2x8 (70% of weight used on week 3)
	Pull Ups	3x6	3x6	3x6	3x6 (70% of weight used on weeks 3)
	Zottman Curls	3x12	3x15	3x15	2x15 (70% of weight used on week 3)
	Planks (30 Sec.)	3x1	3x1	3x1	3x1
Day 3	Deadlift	15x1 (75%; Rest 30 Sec.)	12x1 (80%; Rest 45 Sec.)	10x1 (85%; Rest 75 Sec.)	6x1 (75%; Rest 60 Sec.)
	Sumo Deadlift	2x5 (55%)	2x5 (60%)	2x5 (65%)	2x3 (55%)
	Barbell Bent Over Rows	3x8	3x8	3x6	2x6 (70% of weight used on week 3)
	Barbell Shrugs	3x12	3x12	3x12	2x12 (70% of weight used on week 3)
	Neutral Grip Pull Ups	3x10	3x8	3x6	3x6
	Glute Ham Raises	3x6	3x6	3x6	3x6
	Close Grip Bench Press w/ Resistance Bands	6x3 (60%; Rest 60 Sec.)	6x3 (65%; Rest 60 Sec.)	6x3 (70%; Rest 60 Sec.)	OFF

		8 Week Plan			
		Weeks 5-8			
Day	Exercise	Sets/Reps	Sets/Reps	Sets/Reps	Sets/Reps
		Week 5	Week 6	Week 7	Week 8/Deload
Day 1	Barbell Squat	5x2 (90%; Rest 120 Sec.)	4x2 (95%; Rest 120 Sec.)	2x1 (105%; Rest 120 Sec.)	3x3 (65%; Rest 60 Sec.)
	Pause Squats	3x3 (70%)	3x3 (75%)	3x3 (80%)	3x3 (55%)
	Dead Squats	6x1 (65%; Rest 45 Sec.)	6x1 (70%; Rest 60 Sec.)	6x1 (75%; Rest 60 Sec.)	OFF
	Bulgarian DB Squats	3x8	3x6	3x6	3x3 (70% of weight used on week 7)
	Glute Ham Raises	3x6	3x6	3x6	3x6
	Land Mines	3x8	3x8	3x8	2x8 (70% of weight used on week 7)
	Standing Weighted Crunches	3x12	3x10	3x10	2x10 (70% of weight used on week 7)
Day 2	Bench Press w/ Resistance Bands	Off	1RM	Off	Off
	Dead Bench Press	Off	Off	1RM	Off
	Bench Press	6x3 (85%; Rest 120 Sec.)	6x4 (75%; Rest 60 Sec.)	6x4 (80%; Rest 60 Sec.)	6x3 (60%; Rest 60 Sec.)
	Standing Overhead Press	6x2 (85%; Rest 90 Sec.)	6x2 (85%; Rest 90 Sec.)	6x2 (85%; Rest 90 Sec.)	3x3 (55%; Rest 60 Sec.)
	Close Grip Floor Press	3x6	3x6	3x6	2x6 (70% of weight used on weeks 7)
	Pull Ups	3x6	3x6	3x6	2x6 (70% of weight used on week 7)
	Reverse Barbell Curl	3x12	3x15	3x15	2x15 (70% of weight used on week 3)
Day 3	Deadlift w/ Resistance Bands	1RM	Off	Off	Off
	Deadlift	4x1 (90%; Rest 120 Sec.)	4x1 (95%; Rest 150 Sec.)	2x1 (105%; Rest 180 Sec.)	6x1 (60%; Rest 60 Sec.)
	Deficit Deadlift	Off	10x1 (60%; Rest 45 Sec.)	10x1 (70%; Rest 45 Sec.)	Off
	One-Arm DB Row	3x8	3x8	3x8	2x8 (70% of weight used on week 7)
	DB Shrugs	3x12	3x12	3x12	2x12 (70% of weight used on week 7)
	Neutral Grip Pull Ups	3x6 (Max Weight)	3x5 (Max Weight)	3x5 (Max Weight)	3x5 (70% of weight used on week 7)
	One Leg DB Deadlifts	6x3 (60%; Rest 60 Sec.)	6x3 (65%; Rest 60 Sec.)	6x3 (70%; Rest 60 Sec.)	OFF
	Close Grip Incline Press	3x6	3x5	3x5	3x5 (70% of weight used on week 7)

Some Guidelines to Follow

- Establish legitimate one-rep maxes before starting the program
- Advanced lifters start with 95 percent of true one-rep maxes
- For pull-ups, do band-assisted if you are unable to complete the prescription
- For pistol squats, hold onto a squat rack using a full range of motion if you cannot complete prescription
- For Band Maxes use 10-20% band tension of your 1 rep max, a 400 pound deadlifter would use between 40 and 80 pounds of tension.

Time to hit the pig iron!

12-Week Explosive Strength Makeover

On the field of play, the determining factors between the all-stars and those picking splinters out of their ass from riding the pine are speed and power.

For the no-longer-competitive sportsman, possessing power can mean reigning victorious in any situation; from a self-preservation situation at the local kick n' stab, to a gold medal at the next dwarf-tossing competition.

Power simply means the ability to develop force rapidly. Developing high amounts of force slowly is great for powerlifting… but not much else.

This program is all about creating a more powerful you!

It is important to note that if you are not technically proficient in the Olympic lifts, you should not do this program.

Guidelines

When weights are not given for accessory movements, the instructions are simple: go as heavy as possible without sacrificing technique and completing the allocated number of reps. On dips and pull-ups, add weight if applicable.

If specified weights feel too light, move the weight faster. DON'T add weight to the bar, and DON'T do extra reps.

Remember, moving the bar faster creates higher amounts of force and power.

12 Week Power Program

Week 1

Day 1	Weight %	REPS	SETS	Day 2	Weight %	REPS	SETS
Clean	70,72,75,72,75,77	5,3,1,5,3,1	6	Bench	80	3	3
Low Hang Clean	60	5	3	Speed Bench	70	5	3
Front Squat	72	5	5	Push Press	75	5	5
Pendlay Row		5	3	DB Incline		5	3
RDL		8	3	Tricep Extensions		8	3
Day 3	**Weight %**	**REPS**	**SETS**	**Day 4**	**Weight %**	**REPS**	**SETS**
Snatch	70,72,75,72,75,77	5,3,1,5,3,1	6	Deadlift	70	1	6
High Hang Snatch	60	5	3	Power Clean	60	5	3
Back Squat	82	3	3	Power Snatch	60	5	3
Speed Squat	70	4	6				
Step Ups		16 (8 each leg)	3				

Week 2

Day 1	Weight %	REPS	SETS	Day 2	Weight %	REPS	SETS
Clean	72,75,77,75,77,80	5,3,1,5,3,1	6	Bench	82	3	2
Low Hang Clean	62	5	3	Speed Bench	70	4	8
Front Squat	75	5	5	Push Press	77	5	5
Pendlay Row		5	3	DB Incline		5	3
RDL		8	3	Tricep Extensions		8	3
Day 3	**Weight %**	**REPS**	**SETS**	**Day 4**	**Weight %**	**REPS**	**SETS**
Snatch	72,75,77,75,77,80	5,3,1,5,3,1	6	Deadlift	70	1	6
High Hang Snatch	62	5	3	Power Clean	65	5	3
Back Squat	85	3	2	Power Snatch	65	5	3
Speed Squat	70	4	8				
Step Ups		16 (8 each leg)	3				

Week 3

Day 1	Weight %	REPS	SETS	Day 2	Weight %	REPS	SETS
Clean	75,77,80,77,80,82	5,3,1,5,3,1	6	Bench	85	3	1
Low Hang Clean	65	5	3	Speed Bench	70	4	10
Front Squat	77	5	5	Push Press	80	5	5
Pendlay Row		5	3	DB Incline		5	3
RDL		8	3	Tricep Extensions		8	3
Day 3	**Weight %**	**REPS**	**SETS**	**Day 4**	**Weight %**	**REPS**	**SETS**
Snatch	75,77,80,77,80,82	5,3,1,5,3,1	6	Deadlift	83	5,4,3,2,1	5
High Hang Snatch	65	5	3	Power Clean	65	5	3
Back Squat	87	3	2	Power Snatch	65	5	3
Speed Squat	70	4	10				
Step Ups		16 (8 each leg)	3				

Week 4 Deload Do 3x5 at 60% of Week 3

Week 5							
Day 1	Weight %	REPS	SETS	Day 2	Weight %	REPS	SETS
Clean	80,82,85,82,85,87	5,3,1,3,2,1	6	Bench	87	2	3
Clean Pulls	95 (of full Clean)	3	3	Speed Bench	75	3	6
Front Squat	80	4	4	Push Press	82	3	4
Neutral Grip Pull-Ups	Heavy as Possible	5	4	Seated Military DB Press		8	4
GHR		6	3	Dips		6--10	3
Day 3	Weight %	REPS	SETS	Day 4	Weight %	REPS	SETS
Snatch	80,82,85,82,85,87	5,3,1,3,2,1	6	Deadlift	70	1	6
Snatch Pulls	95 (of full Snatch)	3	3	Power Clean	70	4	3
Back Squat	90	3	2	Power Snatch	70	4	3
Speed Squat	75	3	6				

Week 6							
Day 1	Weight %	REPS	SETS	Day 2	Weight %	REPS	SETS
Clean	82,85,87,85,87,90	5,3,1,3,2,1	6	Bench	90	2	2
Clean Pulls	97	3	3	Speed Bench	75	3	8
Front Squat	82	4	4	Push Press	85	3	4
Neutral Grip Pull-Ups	Heavy as Possible	5	4	Seated Military DB Press		8	4
GHR		6	3	Dips		6--10	3
Day 3	Weight %	REPS	SETS	Day 4	Weight %	REPS	SETS
Snatch	82,85,87,85,87,90	5,3,1,3,2,1	6	Deadlift	70	1	6
Snatch Pulls	97	3	3	Power Clean	70	4	3
Back Squat	92	2	2	Power Snatch	70	4	3
Speed Squat	75	3	8				
Step Ups		16 (8 each leg)	3				

Week 7							
Day 1	Weight %	REPS	SETS	Day 2	Weight %	REPS	SETS
Clean	85,87,90,87,90,92	5,3,1,3,2,1	6	Bench	92	2	1
Clean Pulls	100	3	3	Speed Bench	75	3	10
Front Squat	85	4	4	Push Press	87	3	4
Neutral Grip Pull-Ups	Heavy as Possible	5	4	Seated Military DB Press		8	4
GHR		6	3	Dips		5--7	3
Day 3	Weight %	REPS	SETS	Day 4	Weight %	REPS	SETS
Snatch	85,87,90,87,90,92	5,3,1,3,2,1	6	Deadlift	85	5,4,3,2,1	5
Snatch Pulls	100	3	3	Power Clean	70	4	3
Back Squat	95	2	1	Power Snatch	70	4	3
Speed Squat	75	3	10				
Step Ups		16 (8 each leg)	3				

Week 8 Deload Do 3x5 at 60% of Week 7

Week 9							
Day 1	Weight %	REPS	SETS	Day 2	Weight %	REPS	SETS
Clean	87,90,92,90,92,95	3,2,1,2,1,1	6	Bench	95	1	3
Clean Pulls	105	1	3	Speed Bench	80	2	6
Front Squat	90	3	3	Push Press	90	2	4
Wide Grip Pull-Ups	Heavy as Possible	8	3	Dips		3	5--7
GHR		6	3				
Day 3	Weight %	REPS	SETS	Day 4	Weight %	REPS	SETS
Snatch	87,90,92,90,92,95	3,2,1,2,1,1	6	Deadlift	80	1	6
Snatch Pulls	105	1	3	Power Clean	70	3	3
Back Squat	97	3	1	Power Snatch	70	3	3
Speed Squat	80	2	6				

Week 10							
Day 1	Weight %	REPS	SETS	Day 2	Weight %	REPS	SETS
Clean	90,92,95,92,95,97	3,2,1,2,1,1	6	Bench	97.5	1	2
Clean Pulls	107	1	3	Speed Bench	80	2	8
Front Squat	92	3	2	Push Press	92	2	3
Wide Grip Pull-Ups	Heavy as Possible	8	3	Dips		3	5--7
GHR		6	3				
Day 3	Weight %	REPS	SETS	Day 4	Weight %	REPS	SETS
Snatch	90,92,95,92,95,97	3,2,1,2,1,1	6	Deadlift	75	1	6
Snatch Pulls	107	1	3	Power Clean	75	3	3
Back Squat	100	2	1	Power Snatch	75	3	3
Speed Squat	80	2	8				

Week 11 Deload For Next Week Max Outs. Do 3x5 at 60% of Week 10

WEEK 12 - MAX OUT WEEK!

Increased ROM for Increased Gains

Every gym has an egomaniac that lifts way too much weight with way too little range of motion. Once in a while, these cats may pack on a little size but they generally have the aesthetics of a turtle.

By the odd chance one of these clowns ventures outside his side show by performing exercises with a full range of motion and any sizeable amount of weight, make sure the resident "head doctor" is nearby to counsel his emotional wounds from being introduced to strength reality. Furthermore, have an ambulance on hand for being brought to physical reality.

Science Concurs

Studies continually show that greater range of motion produces greater strength gains and greater amounts of muscle hypertrophy.

Using exercises with a longer range of motion ultimately leads to more time under tension and greater amounts of muscle damage, igniting hypertrophy.

History

Mike MacDonald held the world record in the bench press in the 242-pound weight class for close to three decades, and he actually invented a specialty bar with camber in the middle to increase his bench press range of motion. MacDonald, during a phone conversation with me, reiterated over and over that this is what built hellacious pressing power off his chest.

Virtually every great deadlifter in powerlifting history has used extended range of motion deadlifts to increase starting strength off the floor. Many of the greatest squatters have used deep-pause squats, including Ed Coan.

Gustavo Baddell had immaculate hamstring and back development in his heyday and said, *"I do my deadlifts standing on a deadlift platform so I can get a much deeper stretch and a better range of motion."*

Strength athletes have known for decades that increased range of motion movements build starting strength; smart bodybuilders are catching on.

Application

Let's take a look take a look at the top-six extended range-of-motion movements and how to integrate them into your routine.

Back (Deficit Deadlifts)

Perform deficit deadlifts by standing on a 1-3 inch elevated surface. No platform to stand on? No problem! Instead of deadlifting with 45-pound plates, use 25- or 35-pound plates, or use a wider snatch-grip technique. Perform 6-12 reps for hypertrophy, and 1-5 reps for strength

Legs (Olympic Pause Squats)

Instead of using a traditional squat to parallel, try an Olympic pause squat. Use a narrow foot placement with a high bar position and squat as deep as possible, maintaining proper technique, and pause for one second. For hypertrophy perform 5-10 reps and for strength perform 1-5 reps.

Biceps (Incline Dumbbell Curls)

Give incline dumbbell curls a shot instead of traditional barbell curls; emphasize the stretch at the bottom of the movement to increase range of motion. Perform this movement for 8-15 reps. This was a favorite of "The Austrian Oak," Arnold Schwarzenegger.

Triceps (Neutral Grip Dumbbell Triceps Extensions)

For triceps, instead of barbell skull-crushers, try neutral grip dumbbell triceps extensions to the side of the head, emphasizing the stretch. Perform this movement for 8-15 repetitions.

Shoulders (Incline Dumbbell Lateral Raises)

Opt for incline dumbbell lateral raises over traditional lateral raises, emphasizing the stretch at the bottom of the movement. Perform 10-15 repetitions.

Chest (Dumbbell Bench Press)

Bench pressing a barbell limits the range of motion; why not give dumbbell bench press a shot? Instead of focusing on the weight of the dumbbells, focus on the stretch at the bottom of the movement. Perform 8 -12 repetitions.

Final Thoughts

Using extended range of motion movements extends gains in size and strength.

Proceed with caution, however! Do not sacrifice technique to extend range of motion. In other words, if you lack the mobility to get in a good starting position for deadlifts, don't attempt deficit deadlifts! If shoulder pain at the bottom of a bench press is a regular occurrence, don't start implementing cambered-bar bench presses.

Assuming tightness and technique are not issues, extended range of motion can help build super-human levels of strength and pave the way to hypertrophy heaven.

Time to hit the pig iron!

The Once-a-Week Strength Fix for the "Pump n' Poser"

So you have been training your typical bodybuilding splits religiously, with the type of diligence a Belgian Monk uses when he brews his fabled Trappist beers. You have a good physique and people notice; it is clear you train.

While this is all great on the surface, you know you are weak!

The conundrum lies in the fact that you love your current body part split. When you spoke, we listened and came up with a solution. You get to continue your current routine, BUT — drum roll please — we will have one day a week dedicated to strength.

Remember, strength is primarily a function of the central nervous system. On this day we want all of the movements to be controlled on the eccentric, but the concentric MUST be exploded as hard as possible, this is called Compensatory Acceleration Training. Muscles and the CNS know tension and force. Remember high school physics class? Force = Mass x Acceleration.

Too many lifters forget the acceleration part — we want flat-assed nasty speed. Think mind-movement connection, not mind-muscle connection. Perform this routine once a week in addition to your normal body part split.

Once a Week Strength Fix Routine				
Exercise	**Weight**	**Sets**	**Reps**	**Comments**
Squats	80% 1RM	3	3,3,MAX	Rest 3 minutes between sets. The last set can be done for a repetition max if you feel good
Bench Press	80% 1RM	3	3	Rest 3 minutes between sets. The last set can be done for a rest-pause set if you feel good. Meaning do as many reps as possible (one shy of failure) rest 20 seconds, repeat, rest 20 seconds, repeat. (One Rest-Pause Set is 3 mini sets)
Deadlift	85% 1RM	1	5	Rest 2 minutes between sets. Last set can be done for a repetition max if you feel good.

Conditioning—Burn the Fat, Spare the Muscle!

Ever compare the physiques of a world-class distance runner and a sprinter?

The sprinter resembles a Greek Adonis, while the skinny fat distance runner makes Richard Simmons look like a Mr. Olympia contender.

Adding insult to injury, a 2004 study published in the *Canadian Journal of Applied Physiology* showed rats that performed intense aerobic activity daily experienced not only decreased testosterone levels, but in fact experienced a decrease in the size of the testicles and even the accompanying junk.

Next time someone says "Let's go for a jog," let that person know you cannot afford the shrinkage.

Excessive aerobic activity can decrease testosterone levels, increase cortisol production, weaken the immune system, handicap strength gains, and turn your happy hypertrophy journey into one of catabolism and calamity.

For this reason, many lifters that desire to get big and strong avoid any form of conditioning like the plague.

This is a mistake!

Interval Training Arrival

Since the mid-1990s, scores of studies have shown the effectiveness of interval conditioning for fat loss. In 1994, a Canadian study compared the fat-loss effect of an interval training and traditional, long, slow-cardio regimen. The traditional regimen burned twice as many calories as the interval regimen, but those that performed intervals lost significantly more body fat.

Researchers concluded that "When the difference in the total energy cost of the program was taken into account... the subcutaneous fat loss was nine-fold greater in the HIIT (interval training) program than in the ET (endurance training) program."

Different forms of Tabata intervals are practiced in the most plush commercial gym settings as well as the most Spartan, hardcore gyms in the world. The Tabata regimen consists of performing an activity all-out for 20 seconds, resting 10 seconds and repeating this sequence for four minutes.

Tabata intervals are named after Japanese researcher Izumi Tabata, who has conducted extensive research on interval training.

One of Tabata's most famous findings demonstrated that a program of 20 seconds of all-out cycling followed by 10 seconds of low-intensity cycling for four minutes was as beneficial as 45 minutes of long, slow cardio.

Science clearly concludes that interval training is superior for fat loss, but Tabata demonstrated subjects performing four minutes of high-intensity interval training had similar increases in V02 max as the subjects training traditional cardio four times a week for 45 minutes.

This study was a game-changer because it decisively showed that positive health benefits derived from traditional aerobic training can be accomplished with high-intensity interval training.

Interval Problems

Muscle hypertrophy is elicited from muscle damage, mechanical tension and metabolic stress.

Intervals harshly invoke all three of these mechanisms! Like intense weight training, interval training holds the keys to building a physique of raw steel and sex appeal, BUT intervals must be afforded the same respect as heavy weight.

The Central Nervous System (CNS) is primarily affected by high-intensity work and takes a minimum of 48 hours to recover; so like lifting heavy pig iron, interval training must be allotted similar recovery time.

Jogging slightly fast then walking fast is not interval training in the true sense validated by science. True interval training — pardon the nomenclature — is balls out.

Everything affects recovery!

From weight training to nutrition/supplementation, or employment situation to personal problems, the mind, body and spirit are not compartmentalized; everything factors into how you recover.

The late Charlie Francis, a famed Canadian sprints coach, described the CNS as a cup of tea: everything in life pours tea into the cup, and once the cup of tea overflows you overtrain.

Remember, the further one advances in training, the more stress training imposes.

An intermediate trainee may be able to do three days a week of interval training, whereas a more advanced lifter may only be able to do 1–2 days a week or none at all; high-intensity, high-volume strength training with short rest intervals (how most bodybuilders train) is interval training in itself.

Remember, training adaptations are a consolidated summation of all imposed stressors, both inside the gym and outside.

Applied Interval Training

Training intervals once a week can improve body composition along with conditioning levels; do not perform these workouts more than three times weekly. Twice a week is a nice sweet spot.

Here are some of our favorite interval workouts we have used on ourselves and our clients for fat loss and conditioning.

Strongman Intervals

If you have access to strongman equipment, use it! Go all-out for a medley of 30-60 seconds and you will learn first-hand why this method is so effective.

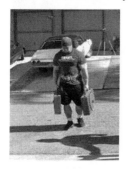

Here are some of our favorite combinations:

Heavy Farmers Walk 50 feet/Heavy Sled Drag 50 feet back. Rest one minute between sets, do as many sets as possible in 10 minutes.

Heavy Yoke 50 feet, Keg Carry 50 feet back. Rest one minute between sets, do as many sets as possible in 10 minutes.

Crucifix Hold 30 seconds, log press with 60 percent of 1 RM x 6 reps. Rest one minute between sets, do as many sets as possible in 10 minutes.

To continually make gains in conditioning and lose pounds of fat, we have to overload our training. To increase intensity with these workouts we have a few different options: increase weight of implements used while still trying to equal previous numbers of sets performed with lighter implements, decrease rest intervals between sets or, of course, just getting more done in the same amount of time.

Ever wonder why strongmen are much leaner than powerlifters? It ain't diet!

Time to hit the pig iron!

Barbell Complexes for Fat Loss

Barbell complexes have been around for decades. Thankfully, in the last decade, there has been a resurgence in this modality that makes body fat run to the hills and takes conditioning to new levels.

Barbell complexes can be done at the end of a strength training workout. They are very easy to implement in your training split.

After leg day, a complex might consist of:

Squats
Good Mornings
Front Squats
Zerchers Squats
Romanian Deadlifts

Barbell complexes are not meant to be paced! Each rep is performed explosively; the objective of the complex is to get each group of exercises done as fast as possible.

Barbell Complex Guidelines:

- Use whole body movements
- Perform exercises fast
- Do not rest between exercises
- Do not drop the bar
- Start with an empty bar and add weights in increments of five pounds
- Barbell complexes are intense interval workouts and are included in your total of interval workouts.

Practical Examples of Barbell Complexes

Complex A

- Back Squat 5-8 reps
- Squat to Push Press 5-8 reps
- Good Morning 5-8 reps
- RDL 5-8 reps
- Bent-Over Rows 5-8 reps
- Power Cleans 5-8 reps

Barbell Complex Progression
Ways to overload barbell complexes:

- Decrease rest intervals
- Increase the weight on the bar
- Increase repetitions per set
- Increase number of sets in same amount of time.

Barbell complexes challenge you mentally and physically… If they are not painful, you are sandbagging!

Start with 5-6 exercises and perform 5-8 reps per exercise. Rest 60-90 seconds between sets and do as many sets as possible in 8-10 minutes.

Burpees

When I think of burpees, an image of a pumped-up convict on a show like "Lock Up" comes to mind. In spite of a horrendous diet and no access to a weight pile, this cat is jacked!

Usually, these men perform burpees like they are going out of style.

Long before burpees were established as a jailhouse favorite, this exercise was a fitness test for the armed services in the World War II era.

Burpees build muscle, burn fat and are one of the most effective conditioning modalities on the planet.

As with the theme of all of our conditioning workouts, we want to keep them less than 10 minutes in total duration.

Total Repetition Method- Select a target number of repetitions; you must hit this number in less than 10 minutes.

If you want 75 burpees, you must do this under 10 minutes. The number of repetitions in a set and the rest interval between sets is at your own discretion. If the objective is 75 burpees in less than 10 minutes, find a way! Stop at 10 minutes regardless of whether you reach 75 burpees or not. If you miss your target, get it next time!

Tabata Burpee Training- Do as many burpees as possible in 20 seconds, rest 10 seconds and repeat this process for four minutes.

To increase intensity with these workouts, we have a couple of different options: increase burpee count (add extra movements to a standard burpee) and increase total number of repetitions.

Walking

Numerous studies have conclusively demonstrated that intense cardiovascular exercise for more 30 minutes at or above 75 percent intensity sabotages strength and hypertrophy gains.

Walking is nowhere near this threshold unless you are severely out of shape. If that's the case, these interval workouts are 100 percent out of the question.

Walking is a great activity to employ on your non-interval conditioning days. You really only need to do a maximum of 30-45 minutes, but even 15-20 minutes will do the job.

Walking benefits:

- Increases General Physical Preparedness (GPP)
- Decreases the Delayed Onset of Muscle Soreness (DOMS) from heavy workouts
- Increases heart health

- Decreases stress
- Helps maintain healthy joints/muscles
- Decreases body fat
- Increases energy levels

Interval training paired with a few weekly walks can help keep you lean and mean while keeping the ticker ticking.

Final Thoughts

Excessive, long, slow cardio destroys strength gains and eats away muscle mass.

Interval training with a couple of weekly walks will improve your health and physique. Interval training is intense; I recommend consulting your physician prior to beginning an interval training program.

No more excuses! You have been given the tools to burn the fat, spare the muscle and improve conditioning.

Time to hit the pig iron!

Less Time = Bigger Results

Tired of all the harassment you receive from friends and family for spending too much time at the gym?

We are going to share with you a method that can cut your gym time in half without sacrificing weight on the bar or quality of work.

Getting more work done in less time simply equals bigger results. Loosely, this idea has spawned the systems of legendary bodybuilding guru and trainer to the stars Vince Gironda. Although he will roll over in his grave when we write this, the late Arthur Jones, while not a high volume guy, advocated maximal intensity in minimal time.

Simply getting more done in less time is called density. When the weight lifted and volume are equal, density trumps longer, drawn-out sessions for strength and size gains every day of the week and twice on Sunday.

Enter Complex Training

Complex training means pairing exercises of two opposing muscle groups or, in scientific terms, an agonist and an antagonist.

Agonists, or "prime movers", are the muscles primarily responsible for generating the force in a specific movement. For a leg extension, the quadriceps is the agonist. An "antagonist" is a muscle that acts opposite to the specific movement generated by the agonist and is responsible for controlling the motion, slowing it down and returning a limb to its initial position. Sticking with the leg extension, the hamstrings serve as an antagonist.

Some examples of exercises that can be paired in a complex format are:

Leg Extensions — Leg Curls
Overhead Press — Pull ups
Triceps Extension — Bicep Curls
Bench Press — Bench Pulls
These are just a few examples! Be creative.

Complex training is being prescribed by more and more strength coaches. Let's not take anybody's word for it — let's see what science has to say.

Science Speaks

A 2009 study published in the *Journal of Sports Sciences* titled "Effects of agonist-antagonist complex resistance training on upper body strength and power development" demonstrates the efficiency of complex training.

Over the course of eight weeks, a group that trained the bench press with bench pulls (an opposing pulling movement for the upper back) improved bench press strength slightly over a group that trained the bench press with traditional sets.

While the complex training group did not have a statistically significant surge in bench press strength over the control group, the study did demonstrate the efficiency of complex training: the same amount of work could basically be done in half the time without compromising strength gains. Demonstrating complex training is an effective means of cutting down time in the gym and continually making gains.

A 2005 study published in the *Journal of Strength and Conditioning Research* entitled "Acute effect on power output of alternating an agonist and antagonist muscle exercise during complex training" suggested that not only does complex save time but it potentially enhances power.

The study found that rugby players with strength-training experience increased power by 4.7 percent when training in the bench press throw as part of a complex with the bench press pull, as opposed to just training the bench press throw by itself. Science says we can save time and not sacrifice strength and power gains from workouts, possibly even enhancing them.

The Lab Meets the Real World

It is important to note most advanced strength athletes do not train this way. The subjects in the aforementioned studies were not competitive lifters. We believe this is because of fatigue. Strength is a product of the Central Nervous System (CNS).

Elite strength athletes have such efficient motor recruitment patterns; in lay terms, they are so skilled at the movements they perform that they fatigue faster. Studies have shown that the stronger an individual is, the longer rest intervals need to be between sets. Remember, we are talking about elite strength athletes, not the vast majority of experienced gym lifters.

If this is you, there are a couple of ways you can handle this. You can continue training with straight sets, as the strongest men in the world have done this for centuries. The second option is what we call modified complex training (MCT). MCT simply means you pair an agonist and antagonist together like complex training.

But here's the kicker!

Place emphasis on one of the movements. If you are capable of doing an overhead press (OHP) of 300 pounds and a pull-up with 80 pounds over your bodyweight for eight reps, emphasizing shoulders might look like this with MCT:

Set 1MCT
OHP 255 Pounds x 5 Reps—Pull-ups Bodyweight x 5 reps
Set 2 MCT
OHP 255 Pounds x 4 Reps—Pull-ups Bodyweight x 5 reps
Set 3 MCT
OHP 255 Pounds x 3 Reps—Pull-ups Bodyweight x 5 reps
The inverse of MCT placing the emphasis on the upper back would look like this
Set 1MCT
Pull-ups 80 Pounds Over Bodyweight x 8 Reps—OHP 155x8
Set 2 MCT
Pull-ups 80 Pounds Over Bodyweight x 6 Reps—OHP 155x8

Set 3 MCT

Pull-ups 80 Pounds Over Bodyweight x 5 Reps—OHP 155x8

This still allows extra stimulation of the antagonist muscle group, without annihilating it.

Final Thoughts

Complex training is the ultimate method to increase training density. If time is of the essence or if you just are looking to try something new — give complex training a shot!

Time to hit the pig iron!

8-Week Olympic Lifting Volume Routine

With the increasing popularity of Crossfit, the Olympic lifts have experienced a resurgence recently… that's the good!

The bad and the ugly are the "armchair" Olympic lifting experts popping up like pills at a Charlie Sheen party. These keyboard warriors have more experience cleaning the porcelain throne than a barbell. Traditionally, it was a rule that you kept the volume relatively low in the classic lifts (the snatch and clean). Today, we see people doing rep maxes in these lifts. This not only undermines the intended purpose of using the Olympic lifts (force-production and speed), but it also puts the athlete at much greater risk for injury.

The Olympic lifts, being as technical as they are, require attention to detail and a relatively "fresh" body. When the body gets too fatigued, the first thing to break down is proper technique.

You might see the butt shoot up out of the bottom of the lift or a rounding of the back during the first pull. Both of these are big no-no's in the Olympic lifts and will invariably end in a missed lift, or worse, becoming acquainted with the local orthopedic surgeon.

A rule of thumb for the people we train is that the highest reps ever done in a set of clean or snatch is six. This includes a small "repositioning" rest (10-20 sec.) between each rep. After six reps, the fatigue you are experiencing can put you out of position. This puts you at risk for injury and also reinforces bad positions that can become habits if done too often.

Don't get us wrong — volume does have its place in a properly periodized Olympic lifting program, especially in the beginning phases of your accumulation cycle where the goal is hypertrophy and building a base for future training.

There are many ways to achieve this volume without performing high-rep cleans and snatches. One of the most effective ways to get the volume needed is by doing complexes.

A complex is basically the use of two or more lifts in conjunction with each other to create one set. Complexes can be used as a low-rep set to work on your weaknesses, but for the purposes of this publication, we are talking about complexes being used as way to achieve some volume in your Olympic lifting workouts.

A sample volume complex could be four hang snatches followed by four overhead squats, or perhaps five cleans followed by five front squats. You want to perform the more technical lift first followed by a lift that is not as technical so that it can be performed correctly while your body is fatigued.

There are so many combinations of lifts that can make up your complexes; this is where your knowledge of your body and its weaknesses comes in. If you are strong from the second pull to the catch but have trouble squatting out your cleans, then you need to work on your leg strength. If your second pull is your problem but you can squat a house, your complex should reflect that.

If your overhead position in the snatch is not rock solid, you could do four hang snatches followed by four overhead pause squats; pausing on the bottom of the overhead squat will help reinforce your catch position. You can't pause an overhead squat without being in a balanced position!

The programming of complexes into your training requires knowledge of your strengths and weaknesses, but a simple 8-week cycle would look something like this. This should be done early in your training cycle where you are primarily concerned with hypertrophy and building a base for training later on down the road.

	Day 1	Day 2	Day 3	Day 4
Weightlifting Complexes				
Week 1-3	(5 Hang Clean-5 Front Squat) x4	(5 Snatch Pull-5 overhead pause squat) x 4	(5 Hang Clean-5 Front Squat) x4	(5 Snatch Pull-5 overhead pause squat) x 4
Week 4 (deload)	(5 Hang Clean-5 Front Squat) x2 @ 60% of week 3	Active Rest	(5 Snatch Pull-5 overhead pause squat) x 2 @ 60% of week 3	Active Rest
Week 5-8	(3 Clean Deadlift - 2 Clean -2 Front Squat) x 4	(2 Snatch DL - 2 hang snatch-4overhead squats) x 4	(3 Clean Deadlift - 2 Clean -2 Front Squat) x 4	(2 Snatch DL - 2 hang snatch-4overhead squats) x 4

Final Thoughts

These complexes should be done with the same weight and directly follow each other. Don't take a break in between the two lifts.

If you are looking to safely add volume to your Olympic lifting program while still working toward the ultimate goal of lifting more weight, give the complex a try.

Time to hit the pig iron!

Supersized Circuit Training

As Charles Dickens once said, *"The pain of parting is nothing to the joy of meeting again."* Similarly, the pain of PHA training is nothing compared to the results it produces.

Peripheral Heart Action Training (PHA) is circuit training on steroids!

This was a favorite cutting strategy of bodybuilders in the 1960s.

We are not talking pink dumbbells or the circuit training at your local *Curves*… this is flat-assed heavy pig iron, but with an extreme conditioning component.

Circuit Training

It is absolutely baffling that circuit training is done primarily on machines while sitting down. One of the main objectives of fat-loss based circuit-training centers is burning calories. Sitting down on machines that do the work of your stabilizer muscles presents a small problem because the exercises are much less metabolically demanding, meaning you burn fewer calories.

Let's take a look at a system that does what circuit training hopes to do when it grows up.

PHA History

This system of bodybuilding circuit training was popularized to the masses by Bob Gajda, a Mr. Universe and Mr. America winner in the 1960s. The idea is to keep circulation of blood through the body throughout the entire workout, which is done by attacking the smaller muscles around the heart first, then moving outward.

This system is vigorous and requires continued, intense exercise for a prolonged period of time without any rest. Because of this, the poorly conditioned bodybuilder and the faint of heart will not do well with this training system.

The idea is to use primarily compound movements for efficiency. The goal is to "shunt" blood up and down the body; this is extremely taxing on the cardiovascular system, but the obvious benefits are a reduction in body fat and, of course, improved metabolic rate.

Because each sequential body part is getting adequate rest between each circuit, strength will be conserved allowing close to maximal strength to be exhibited on the sequential bout. Even though your heart will likely beat at over 150 beats per minute throughout the entire workout, this does not give a license to lower weights; if you have the intestinal fortitude, you should still be able to lift heavy on the rested body part.

Here is a PHA Circuit:

Sequence 1
Standing Dumbbell presses-8-10 reps
Leg raises-10-15 reps
Bent-Over Rows-8-10 reps

Front Squats-5-6 reps
Repeat this sequence three times.

Sequence 2
Weighted dips-8-10 reps
Chin Ups-8-10 reps
Squats-10-12 reps
JM Presses-10-12 reps
Gironda Perfect curls-10-12 reps
Repeat this sequence three times.

Perform the exercises in sequence one for the required number of reps, and do not stop! Repeat the sequence twice more before moving on to sequence two, performing it the same way you did sequence one. Do not rest during a sequence and do not rest between sequences unless absolutely necessary; after all, long breaks defeat the purpose. Maintain your heart rate at 80 percent of your heart rate max; wear a monitor so you can adjust the pace accordingly. If you are in shape, you will not have to trade heavy weight for a slower pace or longer rest.

Variable Manipulation

Doing the same thing over and over and expecting a different result is the definition of insanity!

We are throwing PHA training in the mix to shake things up. I recommend sticking with exercises for the circuits for 3-4 weeks is a row. Each week, however, as you adapt, we need to make the workouts more intense.

The following parameters are how to increase intensity weekly: increase the numbers of reps you have done with the same weight previously, increase the number of sequences (within the same time frame), increase weight on the bar, add bands or chains, or do the workouts more often.

Limit Strength

By now, I think y'all realize big lifts produce the biggest results! Traditional circuit training totally bamboozles any sort of hope in gaining or even maintaining limit strength.

With PHA training, however, the mantra of "go heavy or go home" holds true. The difference is that we are talking about free weight compound movements, not the leg spread machine.

Free weight compound exercises are the most energy-demanding movements in the weight room. These are simply multi-joint movements that necessitate several different muscle groups to work together to the lift the weight; examples are pull-ups, overhead press, dips, squats, deadlifts and bench presses.

These movements burn more fuel because they involve more muscles and allow heavier weights to be used. Want proof of what's harder? Go do a max set of 20 in the deadlift, and then try the same thing with triceps pushdowns.

Heavy free weight multi-joint exercises furthermore serve as a catalyst to the production of good hormones like testosterone and growth hormone. Even if in a "cutting " phase, compound free weight movements cannot be placed in a subservient role — they are your base.

Compound movements have to be the mainstay of PHA training. As long as you are in good shape, you still have to train heavy.

Final Thoughts

PHA training is not as popular because personal trainers would have terrible client retention rates due the sheer pain clients experience; no famous personal trainer or Internet personality makes money because you do PHA training. PHA training benefits just you.

Before illegal anabolic drugs hi-jacked many sound training principles and systems, PHA training helped construct many championship-caliber, lean and muscular physiques.

PHA training is for advanced trainees with a sufficient limit strength base and conditioning levels.

Time to hit the pig iron!

Posing for Size & Strength

Getting maximal results with minimal equipment is a fascinating subject. Where there is a will, there is a way! Being locked in solitary confinement, strapped in a strait-jacket or in any dire situation in between will not exclude you from the benefits of posing.

Anecdotally Supported

Arnold Schwarzenegger believed that by constantly practicing posing he was doing much more than enhancing his stage presence. "The Austrian Oak" believed posing contributed to greater muscular development and even enhanced his ability to throw around heavy pig iron.

Schwarzenegger posed in between workouts, between sets and pretty much any time he wasn't lifting.

Metroflex Gym is the most famous hardcore gym in the world. Not surprisingly, it is home to a wide array of colorful characters that make a Juggalo convention look dull.

One of the most outspoken, entertaining members is a Master's competitive bodybuilder; he is always harping on the fact that one of the most important ways to "harden" up for a show is a daily posing session.

Many consider the late Dr. Mel Siff's book *Supertraining* to be canonical scripture when it comes to the science of strength training. Siff discusses bodybuilding posing and refers to it as, "load less training" and writes about Russians using "load less training" to strengthen muscles and connective tissue.

It seems logical, and certainly anecdotes seem to agree that posing can enhance strength and muscle hypertrophy.

Bro Science to Sound Science

Recently, the Department of Sports and Life Science at the National Institute of Fitness and Sports in Kanoya, Japan, moved this idea from logical speculation to sound science.[1]

The researchers recruited 16 subjects in their early 20s who were in good physical condition. Subjects were divided into a training group of nine people and an inactive group of seven subjects. Over the course of 12 weeks, the training group trained thrice weekly and performed maximal co-contractions of the biceps and the triceps.

In those 12 weeks, the subjects in the training group participated in a 12-week training program with maximal voluntary co-contraction of the biceps and triceps of the right arm three times per week. Basically, with the elbow joint bent to 90 degrees and a neutral forearm position, subjects contracted as forcefully as possible with the biceps and triceps

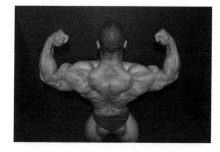

---

[1] Maeo, S., Yoshitake, Y., Takai, Y., Fukunaga, T., & Kanehisa, H. (2013). Neuromuscular adaptations following 12-week maximal voluntary co-contraction training. European Journal of Applied Physiology, 1-11.

for four seconds, followed by a four-second relaxation. This was done 10 times per set and five sets were performed per session, with a two-minute rest interval between sets.

The results were amazing.

The training group significantly increased in strength levels in both the biceps and triceps! Both biceps and triceps significantly increased in size. The functional antagonist muscle relationship between the biceps and triceps was not altered.

Take-home point — posing can build power and prowess.

Practically Applied

Posing helps develop a connection between the mind and the muscle. Including posing habitually in one's training regimen will allow the more efficient contraction of muscles with maximal force; furthermore, what is called "muscle intention" or purposefully contracting the muscle you are training, will be enhanced by posing.

Peak Contraction Enhanced

Bodybuilders love to talk about peak contraction training.

When performing a bicep curl with a peak contraction style, the bodybuilder generally holds the top contracted position for .5 to 1 seconds, squeezing the biceps as hard as possible. Now hit a front double biceps pose flexing as hard as possible for five seconds, and you have just increased time under maximal tension by tenfold!!

Final Thoughts

No one has ever gotten big by posing alone!

Choosing between strength training and posing to maximize muscularity is a no brainer — hit the weights.

To maximally develop a muscle, however, requires a holistic approach with a variety of rep ranges, tempos, intensity levels and contraction types.

At the end of your next arms workout, allocate 10 minutes for a finisher. Contract or "flex" the muscle you trained as hard as possible for five seconds, rest for five seconds. Do this for 10 reps, rest two minutes; do this for 3 sets. We are doing less because we worked out first.

If you want to try this in a separate session, give it a go for 15-20 minutes. Remember, this is not exactly bodybuilding posing. Pose as hard as possible, and if it requires making a nasty face to contract harder...... do it!

This applies to any body part you train.

Posing builds power and physical prowess.

Time to hit the pig iron!

Squats
And
Legs

20-Rep Squats

1896 was a very important year in the strength-training game. This year marked the birth of weightlifting pioneer Mark Berry.

Berry was very successful in his own right, winning a national championship in Olympic weightlifting and becoming the first ever Olympic Games Weightlifting Coach for the United States in 1932 and 1936.

Berry's legacy, however, runs much deeper than personal achievement.

Berry mentored John Grimek, whom many consider the father of modern bodybuilding. Berry, furthermore, immortalized his iron-game legacy with the pen, authoring numerous strength training articles and mail-order courses. He was the first to preach squats for muscular bulk and development. To this day, Berry's teachings help and inspire folks in the iron game.

Arrival of Hise

One inspired pupil was J.C. Hise.

Hise was an all-around badass, always working the toughest types of jobs in coal mines, uranium mills, cement mills, lumber stacking and, as a hobby and in the hope of striking it rich, searching out lost mines and attempting to stake his own claims.

In the early 1930s, Hise commenced barbell training. Using the standard issue routines of the day, J.C. bulked up from 160 to 200 then flat lined at 200. Hise wanted more!

Hise became infatuated with the teachings of Mark Berry after discovering some of his articles advocating the "deep knee-bend" (the modern day squat).

Designing a routine off of Berry's principles, Hise would perform behind the neck presses for 15 reps, full squats for 8 reps, rest, then do 8 more reps. He would then remove 100 pounds from the barbell and do a "balls to the wall" set of 20 reps.

After 30 days, Hise gained 28 pounds from the aforementioned routine, with all muscular measurements significantly improved. This was in conjunction with a high protein diet and copious amounts of milk consumption.

Hise wrote Mark Berry and told him of his success. J.C. was an instant celebrity within the small, but growing, fringe of weightlifters around the US.

Program Evolution

Hise kept on squatting! His program eventually became one all-out set of 20 repetitions. Over time, he morphed into a 298-pound behemoth with a 56-inch chest and 33-inch thighs.

This was long before steroids surfaced. Hise advised eating meat minimally twice daily and drinking plenty of milk.

Legend Grows

As the legend of Hise grew, so did the number of detractors that called "hog wash" on his alleged gains. Many folks travelled across the country to make sure Hise's gains were real, and they were. Naysayers of the 20-rep squat training left Hise as converts.

Over time, legions of men were using the methods Hise had developed from the influence of Mark Berry.

Some iron-game notables, including legendary hard gainer and Ironman Magazine founder Peary Rader, gained 75 pounds after reading about Hise. There were dozens of others, including bodybuilding guru John McCullum.

Nearly 40 years ago Rader said, *"One of the fastest ways to gain size and strength in the entire body is by following the squats and milk program. This is an old time routine that has been around for over 50 years, but it works awesome for fast gains. Even if you are a hard gainer."*

Exercise	Sets	Reps	Comments
The 20 Rep Squat Routine			
Full Squat	1	20	Do 2-3 warm-up sets. For the big work set take a weight you believe you can do 10-12 reps with. For each rep take a couple large mouthfuls of air, hold your breath, squat down ass to grass, repeat. As the set goes on, you will need more and more breaths between reps. Toward the end, you may need five big breaths between reps, that's great! Keep breathing and you will be surprised how long you can keep squatting. Sets can take 2-3 minutes to complete!
Pullovers	1	20	Immediately after squats, grab a light dumbbell and do pullovers on a flat bench. No more than 30 pounds is needed, think stretch in the intercostals (which will give the illusion of a huge chest when fully developed), perform pullovers on a flat bench. Rest two minutes then move on to the Overhead Press.
Standing Overhead Press	3	8	Perform overhead presses standing. Start with your eight-repetition max. Between sets, rest for two minutes, lowering weight in each successive set as needed. Each set should be at or approaching momentary muscular failure. Take a two-minute rest interval before moving onto weighted dips.
Weighted Dips	3	12	Perform weighted dips to a depth of upper arms being parallel to the floor. Start with your 12-repetition max. Between sets, rest for two minutes, lowering weight in each successive set as needed. Each set should be at or approaching momentary muscular failure. Take a one-minute rest interval before moving onto Bent Over Rows.
Bent Over Rows	3	15	Perform Bent Over Rows standing. Torso angle should be between parallel and 45 degrees. A slight cheat is okay toward the end of the set. Start with your 15-repetition max. Between sets, rest for two minutes, lowering weight in each successive set as needed. Each set should be at or approaching momentary muscular failure. Take a two-minute rest interval before moving onto stiff leg deadlift.
Stiff Leg Deadlift	1	15	Stiff Leg Deadlifts are performed standing on a 3-inch block with no weightlifting belt. Keep knees soft as in a 5 to 10 degree bend; bend at the waist keeping the back flat, going as deep as possible without losing this position. One set all-out for 15 repetitions approaching momentary muscular failure.
Pullovers	1	20	Pullovers see note above.

Final Thoughts

There are many variations of the 20-rep squat routine. I tried to pick and choose from these routines as well use my own input and keep in the spirit of Mark Berry and J.C. Hise.

These routines are flat-assed brutal and painful!

Perform this routine twice a week for bulking. If you are paranoid about the lack of bodybuilding movements, go in on a third day and perform isolation movements in a peak contraction style.

Lift hard, eat big, and grow!

Time to hit the pig iron!

■ ■ ■
Low on Time, High on Results — Leg Workout

We are going to do an abbreviated leg workout. Do not view this as a training concession; many legends of iron have thrived on abbreviated workouts. These legends include, but are not limited to, Mike & Ray Mentzer, Dr. Ken Leistner, Dorian Yates, Casey Viator and Boyer Coe.

Science routinely validates the need for higher volume protocols to maximize muscle growth. The question is, how did the aforementioned iron-game iconoclasts get the job done? The answer is intensity! Giving 100 percent and pushing themselves to the limit was the game-changer.

Training with bigger balls requires smaller amounts of volume to catalyze muscle growth.

To get the desired results from the following regimen, you must give 100 percent. In the words of English Philosopher Thomas Hobbes, these workouts will be "nasty, brutish, and short."

Abbreviated Leg Workout			
Exercise	**Sets**	**Reps**	**Comment**
Squats	3	MAX	If you don't have the squat in your program, you don't know squat about leg training! Squats will be performed with a full range of motion. Start with 85 percent of your one-repetition max, do as many reps as possible without failing or having a technique breakdown. Next, do the same thing with 80 percent of your one-repetition max; finally, finish off with 75 percent of your one-repetition max, following the same guidelines. Take a one-minute rest interval between sets and rest three minutes before commencing keystone deadlifts.
Keystone Deadlifts	1	12	Keystone deadlifts are one of the most underrated, underutilized hamstring exercises in existence. We will do one set of 12 reps going as heavy as possible without sacrificing technique.
Bodyweight Squat	1	Juarez Valley 20	So, why not leg extensions to torch the quads? Bodyweight squats are more functional; furthermore, many of our trainees, in the words of Brooks Kubik, are "cellar dwellers" or "garage gorillas", meaning they train at home and may only have access to a barbell and a squat rack. This will not compromise results!

Keystone Deadlifts

The position you assume resembles that of the old time "Keystone Cops," with your butt and belly protruding (lower back is arched). This position causes your hamstrings (back of thigh) to become pre-stretched. Then, while keeping your back arched, lower the barbell down your legs until they reach your knees and stand back up.

Exercise Performance

1. Grab a barbell and stand in an upright position.
2. Bend the knees slightly and keep the shins vertical, hips back and back straight. This will be your starting position.
3. Keeping your back and arms completely straight at all times, push your butt back and bend at the waist.
4. Lower the barbell by pushing the hips back, only slightly bending the knees; think a hinge, not a squat. The barbell remains in contact with your thighs the entire movement.
5. Lower the barbell to just right below the knees.
6. Extend hips back to the starting point.
7. Repeat for prescribed number of repetitions.

Juarez Valley 20 Instructions

Bodyweight squats force one to sit down rather than back, really placing a very intense overload on the quads when contrasted to power squats, not to mention the fact they are a helluva lot more functional than leg extensions.

We will do these in a Juarez Valley 20 format.

The Juarez Valley Method is a creation of the Jailhouse Strong training system. The Juarez Valley Method offers alternating ascending and descending reps. Repetitions are performed in descending order on all odd-number sets, but repetitions are performed in ascending order on even-number sets. In the middle, they meet! A Juarez Valley 20 is performed liked this:

Set 1 - 20 reps
Set 2 - 1 rep
Set 3 - 19 reps
Set 4 - 2 reps
Set 5 - 18 reps
Set 6 - 3 reps
Set 7 - 17 reps
Set 8 - 4 reps
Set 9 - 16 reps
Set 10 - 5 reps
Set 11 - 15 reps
Set 12 - 6 reps
Set 13 - 14 reps
Set 14 - 7 reps
Set 15 - 13 reps
Set 16 -8 reps

Set 17 - 12 reps
Set 18 - 9 reps
Set 19 - 11 reps
Set 20 - 10 reps

Between each set, the rest interval is an eight-foot walk across your "cell" or wherever you train. The goal is to complete this sequence in less than eight minutes. Keep track of time, and continually strive to beat previous time records as opposed to adding sets.

Final Thoughts

With very little time and maximum intensity, great results can be accomplished. Do not compromise results; give this abbreviated routine a try.

Time to hit the pig iron!

Holistic Muscle Building Approach

In the 1930s, weightlifting pioneer JC Hise discovered a mass-building miracle by doing one set of 20 reps all-out in the squat. Perry Reader carried the torch and shared this method with the masses in the 1950s and 60s. Entire books have been written on the 20-rep squat methodology.

To this day, the 20-rep squat method has disciples.

The 5 sets of 5 reps methodology was popularized by Reg Park, Arnold Schwarzenegger's mentor and hero. Park was arguably the best bodybuilder of all time prior to 1960. Bill Starr, world famous strength coach and author, has since advocated 5 sets of 5 reps, as did Mark Henry and Brad Gillingham. Bigger Faster Stronger (BFS), a popular high school and college training methodology, has adopted this method at the nucleus of its strength program.

Both methods have die-hard advocates, and both have produced monsters in classical and recent eras.

Who's right?

A recent Japanese study confirmed that when adding a high-repetition set at the end of a 5 x 5 program, hypertrophy gains averaged eight percent better than just doing the 5 x 5 alone. Furthermore, greater strength gains were induced with inclusion of a high-rep back-off set and the acute growth hormone response was greater.

The researchers concluded: "The results suggest that a combination of high- and low-intensity regimens is effective for optimizing the strength adaptation of muscle in a periodized training program."[2]

What Does this mean?

A number of old-school bodybuilders and powerlifters advocate a back off set. In other words, after the heavy weight has been lifted on a given exercise, do a high-rep set.

It is important to do the heavy weight first for a couple reasons; after the all-out high rep set, muscular fatigue is induced and the heavy set will allow more reps to be lifted with the subsequent lighter weight. This is a trick that has been used by smart NFL combine specialists for years; warm up to 275 to 315 pounds on the bench press before doing an all-out repetition max at 225.

This works because of Post Activation Potentiation (PAP), meaning the heavy lift allows one to produce more force on the subsequent light set.

---

[2] Goto, K., Nagasawa, M., Yanagisawa, O., Kizuka, T., Ishii, N., & Takamatsu, K. (2004). Muscular Adaptations To Combinations Of High- And Low-Intensity Resistance Exercises. *Journal of Strength and Conditioning Research*, *18*(4), 730-737.

The Workout

Holistic Approach				
Exercise	Sets	Reps	Rest	Comment
Squats	5	5	3-4 Min	Start light, second set should increase in weight, third set should be your top weight. Try and maintain that weight for the remaining two sets.
Squats	1	20		Use a weight you normally can do 12-15 reps with. Take 2-3 deep breaths between reps when it feels like you are close to failing. Keep pushing you will make it
Leg Extension	3	12,12,40	1 Min	Maximum intensity without sacrificing form
Nordic Leg Curls	3	4	1 Min	5 second eccentric

Final Thoughts

Fred Hatfield was right over 30 years ago: fully developing a muscle requires a holistic approach that requires a wide variety of rep ranges.

Real science has confirmed what in-the-trenches bro science has said for decades.

Time to hit the pig iron!

The All-Dumbbells Leg Mass Plan

Exercise fads are here and gone in a New York minute!

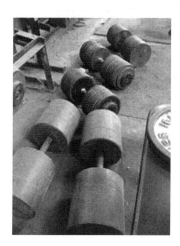

In 200 A.D. Galen, a Greek physician, wrote a text detailing the virtues of dumbbell training and the healing benefits of training with dumbbells. Not a whole helluva lot has changed!

Any exercise scientist or iron-game aficionado knows nothing beats a pair of dumbbells for price, simplicity, and most importantly, results.

Let's look at a routine to build a massive set of wheels with nothing required but dumbbells.

The following three exercises are performed in a giant set; we will do a set of five reps, a set of 15 reps and a set of 40 reps, done without rest between sets. Furthermore, there is no rest between giant sets. This means you will be doing 130 reps in a row with no rest.

Of course, you can take time to change dumbbells and move to a different exercise, but that is a matter of 5-10 seconds. Yes, it can be done! You may need to lower the weight used a bit, but not much.

Giant Set DB Leg Blast			
Exercise	Sets	Reps	Comment
Keystone Deadlifts	1	5	
DB Squats	1	15	Perform This Giant Set Twice With No Rest
DB Lunge	1	40	

Go as heavy as possible while maintaining good form; perform this giant set twice. Make sure you are properly warmed-up so you can give the required 100 percent right off the bat to maximize results.

This workout was inspired by the incomparable Dr. Fred Hatfield.

Time to hit the pig iron!

The Ultimate Quad/Ham Routine

"Remember this: your body is your slave; it works for you"
- Jack LaLanne.

To get the most out of leg day, this needs to be your attitude. We are going to look at the ultimate quad/ham routine, which is applicable to the working professional with limited time in the gym who would still challenge the most seasoned pro.

Squats

Ronnie Coleman, the greatest bodybuilder of all-time, commenced every leg workout with heavy squats. So did Tom Platz, who many consider to have the greatest legs of all time.

Branch Warren fan? Well, he kicks off leg day with squats, too.

Virtually every study performed on squats confirms their efficiency for athletic transference, size, strength and anabolic hormone secretion.

For development, we will be using a full range of motion.

After you are warmed up, you just have to squat for 15 minutes. Start with a weight you are capable of doing 10 reps with. For set one, do seven reps.

Rest one minute and attempt seven reps again; if you are unable to do seven reps do six reps, if you cannot do six reps do five… you can keep this up all the way to set of one. Repeat this process for 15 minutes.

If you feel good on the last set, do as many reps as possible (AMAP).

Leg Curl/Romanian Deadlift /GHR (Giant Set)

The hamstrings have two functions: flexion of the knee and extension of the hips. Romanian deadlifts work primarily hip extension and leg curls work knee flexion. The glute-ham raise attacks both functions in one exercise!

The hamstring is a predominantly fast-twitch muscle and it responds very well to low reps. That's why most bodybuilders have poor hamstring development compared to quads; the best hamstrings are seen on Olympic lifters and sprinters who train explosively in short bursts.

All three exercises will be performed for sets of six reps.

Rest 10 seconds between individual giant-set exercises. The giant set works by attacking all functions of the hamstrings in a fatigued state. The widest pool of motor units will be recruited, catalyzing the biggest increases in hypertrophy.

Rest interval is two minutes between giant sets, for a total of three giant sets. Each one should be as heavy as possible while maintaining great form. You will have to lower weight each giant set.

Sissy Squat — Leg Extension Superset

Sissy squats are a forgotten bodyweight exercise that has contributed to many championship sets of quads! Alone, these are difficult, but supersetted with leg extensions they are real-life quadriceps hades!

For sissy squats, perform 15 repetitions followed immediately by 30 repetitions on the leg extension. Each set of leg extensions should require a maximum effort without sacrificing form.

Do three supersets with a two-minute rest interval between sets.

Ultimate Quad/Ham Routine				
Exercise	Weight	Sets	Reps	Comments
Squats	10RM	AMAP	1--7	Last set Rest-AMAP. Rest 60 seconds between sets. Do not exceed 15 minutes.
Leg Curl-RDL-GHR (Giant Set)	MAX	3	6,6,6	Rest 2 minutes between giant sets, 10 seconds between exercises within giant sets.
Sissy Squat-Leg Extension (Superset)	BW/MAX	3	15-30	Rest 2 minutes between supersets

Final Thoughts

You don't always get what you wish for; you get what you train for! This routine maximizes your results as you give maximum effort.

Time to hit the pig iron!

■ ■ ■
Powerbuilding — Leg Training

Developing serious strength has sucked hind tit for far too long in the regimens of bodybuilding enthusiasts.

The founding fathers of bodybuilding were required to perform feats of strength in addition to their posing routines. Guys with great physiques possessed great strength and power, and guys that possessed great strength and power did not look like the regulars at Golden Corral.

Even if you couldn't care less about lifting heavy weights, realize that your limit strength is your base. Don't get mad at me, I don't make the rules.

Bodybuilders must train core lifts. Strength athletes must include the small exercises that assist in the ultimate performance of core lifts.

Science and anecdotes both concur that a wide volume of intensity and exercises must be included in one's repertoire to maximally develop a muscle.

Legs

There is nothing as silly as seeing chicken legs serving as the base to a massively developed upper body. Thankfully, in the modern era, bodybuilding places a high precedent on lower-body development.

We are going to build your legs, keeping strength at the core of the program.

Powerbuilding Training - Legs

Exercise	s	Reps	Comments
Squats	4	5,4,3,3	"Shut up and squat!" the motivational gym poster says. Start these with a five rep max weight. The objective is to use the same weight for all four sets. Rest 2-4 minutes between sets. All squats should be performed in a low bar power style, slightly below parallel.
Olympic Pause Squats	2	8	Use a high bar placement and a narrow foot placement between shoulder and hip width. Squat with an ass to grass style, without making technique the sacrificial lamb. Pause in the bottom position for one second. The pause will prolong time under tension and eliminate the assistance of the stretch shortening cycle (the elastic-like energy stored on the negative that assists on the way back up of the lift). Go as heavy as possible, rest 2-4 minutes between sets.
Leg Extension 2 Up-1 Down	3	8	Leg Extension (2 up 1 down). Remember, the purpose is isolation of the quads so do not let this become an ego lift by using weights that alter technique or tempo. Pick a weight you can do 12-15 strict repetitions with. Do a leg extension with both legs but remove the leg you are not working at the extended position and lower the weight with the one leg you are working for a count of five seconds. Repeat this seven more times and then switch sides. Eccentric overload work is essential to maximum muscular development. Rest 30 seconds between sides/sets.
Romanian Deadlift	2	6	Romanian Deadlifts-The hamstrings extend the hip and flex the knee. Far too many bodybuilders forget about the hip extension part. We will leave no stone unturned, working the hamstrings hip extension with this tried and true classic. Remember, this is not a straight leg deadlift, keep a slight bend in the knee throughout the movement, push the hips back while lowering the barbell (you should feel tension in the hamstrings), stop when the torso is parallel to the floor, then lift the weight back up by extending the hips. Rest 1-2 minutes between sets.
Leg Curl	3	4	Leg Curls (2 up 1 down). Do not let this become an ego lift by using weights that alter technique or tempo. We are keeping the reps low because hamstrings are primarily a fast-twitch muscle, so in turn, they respond best to lower reps. Pick a weight you can do 8-10 strict repetitions with. Do a lying leg curl with both legs but remove the leg you are not working at the flexed position and lower the weight with the one leg you are working for a count of five seconds. Repeat this three more times then switch sides. Eccentric overload work is essential to maximum muscular development. Rest 30 seconds between sides/sets.
Prison Squats	1	AMAP in 2 Min.	Prison Squats. Prison Squats are just bodyweight squats with your hands held behind your head. Use a shoulder-width stance and squat as deep as possible each rep. Prison squats force you to squat downward more than back, like a power squat, in turn torching the quads. Do as many bodyweight reps as possible in two minutes.

Final Thoughts

Maximum development requires a holistic approach, because that's what powerbuilding is. We are keeping strength fundamentals in the process, synergistically mixing compound movements, tempos and rep schemes.

We are leaving no stone unturned in our journey to hypertrophy heaven.

Time to hit the pig iron!

From Calves to Bulls Listening to Internet banter, training calves is a waste of time. One's parents are the sole factor to great calf development.

How depressing!

Many would have written off the calf development of the "Austrian Oak" Arnold Schwarzenegger. At first glance, it appeared Schwarzenegger was a prisoner of genetics and would never have great calves. Schwarzenegger busted out of his genetic prison sentence and built some of the greatest calves of all-time.

Schwarzenegger made huge sacrifices in pursuit of calf development. While some people feel driving five minutes to the gym is a huge sacrifice, Schwarzenegger moved to South Africa for a summer to train with his idol, Reg Park.

Park trained his calves daily, performing calf raises in excess of 1,000 pounds. Lesson learned! Schwarzenegger, later in his career, was accused of calf implants because of his extreme calf development. He adamantly denies this and there is not a shred of evidence to support the accusation.

The only place where success comes before work is in the dictionary. Development of all muscles does involve a genetic component; anecdotally, even more so with calves. The good news, as learned from Arnold and Reg Park, is that we can train calves heavy and frequently.

When performing the prescribed calf movements keep these four rules in mind:

1. Full range of motion equals full development. DO NOT SACRIFICE RANGE OF MOTION.
2. Control negative portion of the rep, explode the positive. When a specific tempo is prescribed, follow it; sacrifice weight before tempo.
3. Don't bounce calf exercises. Think muscle, not momentum.
4. Go as heavy as possible, adhering to the first three rules.

The prescribed workouts can be added to existing workouts or performed in separate sessions. Training a weak point? Begin the workout with calf work when fresh.

Calf to BULL

Day	Exercise	Sets/Reps	Comments
Day 1	Donkey Calf Raises	5x10	Pause two seconds at the top and two seconds at the bottom. Go as heavy as possible without sacrificing range of motion. 90 seconds between sets.
Day 2	Seated Calf Raises	5x50,40,30,20,10	Use a weight you can do 50 reps with the first set; rest 120 seconds between sets with a goal of using the same weight all five sets without sacrificing technique
Day 3	OFF		
Day 4	Standing Calf Raises (2 Up 1 Down)	5x5	Perform a standing full range of motion calf raise. From the top plantar flexed position, lower yourself to the bottom position, using only one leg with a steady five-second eccentric. Use as much weight as possible; a good starting point is a weight you could comfortably perform 15-20 reps with two legs in a traditional fashion. Rest 2:30 between sets.
Day 5	Banded Tibia Raises	5x30	Leaving no stone unturned, we will be performing band tibia raise which work the Tibialis Focus on keeping the movement strict at the ankle. Rest one to two minutes between sets.
Day 6	Calf Presses on Leg Press	5x15	Go as heavy as possible without sacrificing technique. Rest one to two minutes between sets.
Day 7	OFF		

Final Thoughts

First and foremost, if your calves suck they've gotta become a priority.

A couple half-assed sets at the end of a workout when dead tired will not cut the mustard. Do these exercises fresh, with maximum intensity, following the prescribed guidelines.

Time to hit the pig iron!

Foundational Leg Training

Chicken legs are great for dinner but sure look silly on commercial gym "pec-and-bi warriors!"

If you will give us 45 minutes of your time weekly, we can take your leg development to a whole new level. We are going to do one core exercise, one superset and one bodyweight finisher.

Since we are doing a few exercises for a short period of time, we need 100-percent concentration and focus while training.

Squats

Bodybuilding enthusiasts that debate about the most developed legs of all-time have it narrowed it down to Tom Platz or Branch Warren. Personal opinions aside, the fact remains that both men credit their leg development to heavy, high-volume squats.

Even Ronnie Coleman, the greatest bodybuilder of all-time, commenced every leg workout with heavy squats.

Let's look beyond the functional benefits of the squat. A University of North Dakota study demonstrated that with equivalent loads, the squat worked the glutes and hamstrings significantly more than the leg press and, surprisingly, even the quads.

Scores of studies show squatting produces an enormous spike in anabolic hormones. Squats even train your cardiovascular system because of the hypoxia effect, meaning temporarily, while squatting, oxygen intake is inadequate. Not only does this build a strong heart and lungs but revs up the metabolism, building a key ally in the fat-loss war.

Half squats equal half results!

Check the ego at the door and go full range of motion for full development.

Instead of squatting for hours on end, efficiency is the name of the game. After you are warmed up, you have 12 minutes to complete all squats. Start with a weight you are capable of doing 8-10 reps with. For set one, do five reps.

Rest 60 seconds and attempt five reps again; if you are unable to complete five reps do four, if you cannot do four reps do three, if you cannot do three reps do two, and if two reps is too much, do one. Always stop one shy of failure but do not exceed five repetitions. Repeat this process for 12 minutes. The clock starts once you have completed your first set.

On the last set, if you still have something left, go for an all-out rep max stopping one repetition shy of failure.

When you can complete 40 repetitions in this time period, increase the weight on the bar by five percent; if you cannot, make sure you beat your previous rep record.

Squat Technical Tips:

- Place a barbell on top of the posterior deltoids
- Un-rack the barbell and step back one leg at a time to a shoulder-width or wider stance
- Keep your chest up and shoulder blades retracted
- Initiate movement by pushing your hips back (don't bend at the knees first)
- Make sure to push your knees out on the descent and ascent
- Squat down below parallel
- Return to the starting position

If you still have reservations about squatting, heed the words of the classical squattin' poem by Dale Clark.

Down this road, in a gym far away,
a young man was heard to say,
"no matter what I do, my legs won't grow"
he tried leg extensions, leg curls, and leg presses, too
trying to cheat, these sissy workouts he'd do.

From the corner of the gym where the big men train,
through a cloud of chalk and the midst of pain
where the noise is made with big forty fives,
a deep voice bellowed as he wrapped his knees.
a very big man with legs like trees.

Laughing as he snatched another plate from the stack
chalking his hands and monstrous back,
said, "boy, stop lying and don't say you've forgotten,
the trouble with you is you ain't been SQUATTIN'."

Leg Curl/Romanian Deadlift Superset

The hamstrings have two functions: flexion of the knee and extension of the hips. Romanian deadlifts work primarily hip extension and leg curls work knee flexion. Let's attack both functions in one superset!

With the leg curl, we are going to do a negative overload by curling up with both legs and lowering the weight with one leg for a five-second count. Do this for five reps each side.

How to correctly perform an eccentric one-leg overload leg curl:

- Lie face down on the leg curl; adjust it to fit your body
- Put the pad of the lever slightly below your calves
- Keep your torso flat on the bench
- Grasp handles on the side of the machine
- Make sure your legs are fully stretched and curl your legs up as far as possible
- Hold briefly at the top
- Lower with one leg for a steady five-second count
- Return to the starting position

Important note: Leg curls need to be strict and full range of motion. Start with 25-percent more than what you can do on a concentric (positive) leg curl.

Romanian Deadlifts

Romanian Deadlifts (RDLs) are one of the all-time great hamstring builders. We will be doing RDLs for sets of six reps, as heavy as possible, while maintaining good form.

How to correctly perform a Romanian deadlift:

- Start this movement standing upright
- Take a stance between hip and shoulder width; place your hands outside of your thighs
- Use a pronated grip (straps are okay)
- Slightly bend your knees, and keep your back arched and flat
- Lower the bar, keeping your chest up by pushing your hips back and purposely putting tension on the hamstrings
- Lower the bar to mid-shin level (your torso should be parallel to the floor)
- Lift the weight to the starting position by extending the hips
- Keep the bar in close to your body; the further it drifts away from you, the more stress will be put on your lower back

The reps are low on purpose. Hamstrings are primarily a fast-twitch muscle group and respond best to lower reps. This is why most bodybuilders lag in the hamstrings compared to the quads and why sprinters have the greatest hamstring development of any athlete.

We will do both exercises supersetted followed by a 90-second break for 10 minutes. Do as many supersets as possible in 10 minutes, maintaining good form.

The Finisher

The last exercise of the day is bodyweight squats. These force an athlete to sit more down than back, shifting a greater emphasis onto the quads.

We will do this for a "Jailhouse 20", which is a total of 210 total repetitions, where set 1 is performed with 20 repetitions, set 2 is 19 repetitions, set 3 is 18 repetitions, etc. Each set descends by one less repetition. After each set is performed, walk 16 feet (8 feet across your "cell" and 8 feet back).

Complete the Jailhouse 20 as fast as possible and keep track of time. If it is not complete at eight minutes, stop regardless of where you are.

Foundation Leg Training				
Exercise	**Sets**	**Reps**	**Intensity**	**Rest Interval**
Squats	MAX	1--5	8-10RM	60 Sec.
Eccentric One Leg Overload Leg Curl/RDL	MAX	5--6	MAX	90 Sec.
Bodyweight Squats	20	20--1	Bodyweight	16 Ft. Walk

Final Thoughts

A big house requires a big foundation.

*"The only thing standing between you and the strongest man in the world is
how many times you can put five more pounds on the bar and squat it,"*
-My first powerlifting mentor, Steve Holl.

Time to hit the pig iron!

Power Rack Leg Training

Is your training suffering? Probably because you can never push sets anywhere close to failure or lift heavy enough weights to catalyze serious gains in size and strength because of a lack of spotters and reliable training partners.

Dry your eye — a lack of training partners does not have to mean a lack of results.

Pushing sets to repetition maximums, partial overloads and virtually any strength-building barbell movement can be accomplished in solitude by using the power rack!

Fail with a weight? No big deal, the pins, your "built-in spotters," will allow you to flee to safety.

Except for hotel and corporate chrome-palace chain gyms that have made an effort to round up and run off the "usual suspects" — as in you, the serious lifter — all gyms have power racks.

My advice to you is if a gym does not have a power rack, leave!

Sure, you can get great results without a power rack, but in a roundabout way, this is an attitude of disdain toward serious strength training.

In days past, there would be a fight to train on any available power rack! Nowadays, power racks are collecting dust. While this is unfortunate for the physiques of the masses, it is great for the old heads that train seriously.

In this workout we are going to build some serious size and strength in the power rack.

Go to the gym, park your ass in the power rack and do not leave until the workout is complete. This may not be the best way to win friends, but we are at the gym to get big and strong, not make friends.

Power Rack Leg Routine			
Exercise	**Sets**	**Reps**	**Comments**
Squats	4	3,5,6,12	*Full squats have played an important role of virtually all iron game athletes that possess serious size and strength. Full range of motion is the name game; make sure every squat breaks parallel. Each set should be with limit poundage but not to all-out failure, stopping one rep of shy of true failure. Between sets rest 3-4 minutes*
Front Squats	2	6	*Front squats are a great tool to teach squatting with an upright posture. Bend over with these and lose the weight; good form is a natural byproduct. Many prominent strength coaches feel this squatting variation has the best transfer of training to sports; bodybuilders love this movement because it is more quad dominant than a back squat. Full range of motion is the name game; make sure every front squat breaks parallel. Each set should be with limit poundage but not to all-out failure, stopping one rep of shy of true failure. Between sets rest 3-4 minutes.*
1/2 Dead Squats	1	3	*1/2 Dead Squats are an excellent way to handle overload supramximal weights. If you can do 400 here, next time you squat 300, it will not feel so heavy. Set the loaded barbell on the pins in what would be a half squat position, from the bottom position squat the barbell off the pins to completion like a regular squat. This builds starting strength because of the removal of the negative portion of the lift that allows lifters to store elastic-like energy that aids them in lifting the weight up. Because of the reduced range of motion, heavier weights can be handled. Use progressively heavy weight for each single repetition ending with a one-rep max. Between sets rest 2-3 minutes*
Good Mornings	3	8	*Perform good mornings with great form! If this becomes an ego lift you will get hurt and rob the hamstrings of the work we are after, the squatting variations so far do work the hamstrings but for the overload needed for balanced strength and symmetry, we need to include good mornings. Do not round your back whatsoever, make sure your core is braced and tight. Perform this movement with a slight bend in the knee, go until your torso is parallel to the floor, if you lack mobility stop before you round. Go as heavy possible keeping great technique. Between sets rest 1-2 minutes*
Bodyweight Squats	1	MAX	*Bodyweight squats are a fantastic finisher to torch the quads! Bodyweight squats force one to sit straight down rather than back like a power squat, providing the quads with a huge overload. Perform as many repetitions as possible in 90 seconds for one set using a full range of motion.*

Final Thoughts

If you have a power rack, a barbell, and weights, you have no excuse not to have a great physique and strength levels to match.

The soft culture at commercial gyms opens up available power racks for us to take our training to the next level.

Time to hit the pig iron!

Leg Training — Giant Sets in a Hurry

The following workout can be compared to a ham and egg breakfast; the chicken laid an egg to be part of the breakfast and the pig gave his life to get on the plate. To succeed with this workout, you've gotta be the pig by giving 100 percent.

Giant Sets — What and Why?

A giant set is four or more exercises paired together with minimal rest that target one body part. Done intensely enough, it will even provide cardiovascular benefits. Giant sets cause a spike in production of growth hormone and IGF-1. Giant sets are designed to target the trained muscle at various angles.

Giant sets increase metabolic stress because of the continuous sequence. Because the muscle is hit so hard and at so many different angles, exercise-induced muscle damage results. This is a key element in becoming large and in charge.

Giant sets are associated with marathon workout sessions; think about it logically, if four different exercises are combined with no rest, that's silly.

Move from exercise to exercise as fast as possible. Take a rest interval of five minutes between giant sets (all four exercises).

Giant Sets			
Exercise	**Sets**	**Reps**	**Comments**
Front Squat	2	4	*Many strength coaches consider the front squat their "go to" exercise; numerous bodybuilders credit this exercise with developing shapely, robust quadriceps. Start with your four-rep max, do as many reps as possible (if you can do more than four, keep on trucking). On the second giant set, do the same thing. More than likely you will do fewer reps BUT that doesn't mean less effort, go balls out.*
Back Squat	2	8	*Many times the limiting factor in the back squat is the lower back; with legs pre-fatigued this issue is nearly eliminated. Perform this movement with your eight-repetition max for both sets, if you can do more, do it! If you do less, that's fine, assuming you are giving a full effort.*
2 up - 1 down Leg Curls	2	5	*2-up-1 down Leg Curls is performed on a lying leg curl. Pick the heaviest weight you can possibly handle without sacrificing the tempo. Curl the weight up using the hamstrings with both legs, at the top contracted position release one leg and lower the weight to the starting position, following a strict five-second tempo. Hamstrings are primarily a fast-twitch muscle group so they react really well to lower reps and particularly eccentric overloads.*
Leg Extensions	2	40	*Perform the leg extensions in a slow, rhythmic style; achieving all 40 reps is the purpose, focus on the mind-muscle connection and continuous tensions. Your quads have already handled the heavy pig iron, this is putting on the finishing touches. The leg extensions artificially isolate the quadriceps unlike any normal human movement; this is why we do them. The artificial isolation provides an overload stimulus to the quad, particularly "the sweep."*

Final Thoughts

This is another Fred Hatfield inspired workout, who used a similar approach while working with Lee Haney. Enough talk, time to hit the pig iron!

German Volume Training for Legs

What do Bill Kazmaier and Bev Francis have in common? One is arguably the strongest man to ever walk the face of the earth and the other put female bodybuilding on the map. Also, both trained periodically with 10 sets of 10 reps.

Charles Poliquin, possibly the greatest strength coach of all-time, legendary East German Weightlifting demigod Rolf Fesser, and bodybuilding guru Vince Gironda have all endorsed the 10 sets of 10 method to add muscle mass to athletes.

Because of the success Rolf Fesser had with weightlifters adding mass, Charles Poliquin coined the term German Volume Training (GVT) for the 10 sets of 10 method.

Hell, I used this method in my journey to add mass in the off-season to become the youngest human being to bench press 600 pounds.

High Volume

It's time to quit ridin' the gravy train on biscuit wheels and put in some work!

Make no bones about it, this is a very high volume routine and, more than likely, has Mike Mentzer rolling over in his grave.

Volume is defined as *reps x sets x poundage lifted*. Science and in-the-trenches experience concur that in general, higher volume produces more hypertrophy. That's why compound movements are the method of choice for a ticket to hypertrophy heaven.

Let's look at an example working the quadriceps using the Olympic squat and the leg extension.

If four sets of 10 repetitions are performed on the Olympic squat with 350 pounds, the total volume is 4 x 10 x 350 = 14,000 pounds. If we did the same workout with leg extensions using 60 pounds, the total amount of volume would be 4 x 10 x 50 = 2,000 pounds.

That's seven times more volume with Olympic squats!

Bottom line: a lot more volume can be accomplished with emphasis on compound movements. This is the essence of German Volume Training!

More on GVT

Nowadays, a majority of educated coaches and athletes correctly use compound movements as their bread and butter to slap on size, and after they perform the main barbell movement in a training session, they strive to hit the muscle from all different angles.

This is done with supplementary core lifts (for example, performing a front squat after a back squat) and, of course, multiple sets and repetitions of isolation movements. The objective is to reap the benefits of the core movement and stimulate as many muscle fibers as possible by attacking the muscle from a variety of angles with a number of movements.

GVT Alternative

What's the alternative? Attack the same movement with multiple sets, many more than typically recommended.

Originally, GVT was a protocol of 10 sets of 10 repetitions of a compound movement, using a 20-repetition max, or approximately 60 percent of the athlete's one-rep max. Rest periods of 60 seconds up to three minutes have been advocated; however, rest depends on the movement being performed, the load used, and the anaerobic capacity of the athlete.

In the event of not being able to complete all of the repetitions, reduce the load by 2.5–5 percent; so if you were using 200 pounds and did not complete the final rep on the seventh set, use 190–195 pounds on the following set.

While this reduction is quite minor, we want to keep the intensity as high as possible for maximum muscle growth. If you attempt to keep the weight the same and continually miss reps because of fatigue, you won't reap the intended benefits of GVT.

Think about it.

Performing only five reps on your last set, even if you had made every rep until that point, reduces the total volume of that set by 50 percent! Done over multiple sets, the protocol has been significantly compromised, which destroys the intended training effect. German Volume Training is 10 sets of 10 repetitions. Either get to work or join Planet Fitness.

How Does GVT Work?

Because of the high-volume training load and short rest intervals, this method produces a very anabolic growth hormone response.

The idea, as Poliquin has written, is to attack the same muscle fibers over and over with the same movement for extremely high volume, as this will force the muscle fibers to experience major growth.

German Volume Training Leg Workout

- **1a. Squats: 10x10 (rest 20 seconds before 1b start 60 percent of one-rep max)**
- **1b. Leg Curls: 10 x 10 (rest three minutes before repeating complex; if bodyweight becomes too difficult, go band-assisted)**

Final Thoughts

Besides muscle hypertrophy, German Volume Training can benefit the cardiovascular system. One study on professional rugby players performing a GVT bench press routine showed that by their last set, their heart rates climbed to 160 beats per minute and never dropped below 120 during the recovery phase. Imagine that with squat!

Even if you are pressed for time, following the rest periods exactly, this workout will take under an hour.

German Volume Training requires big balls but yields big results!

Time to hit the pig iron!

DEADLIFT AND BACK

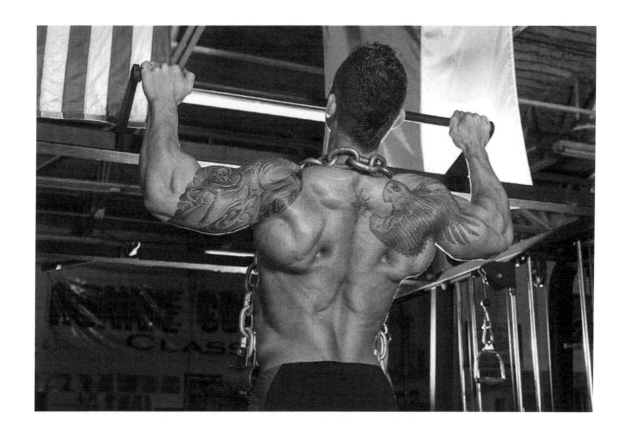

■ ■ ■
The Deadlift Encyclopedia

Pick up your kid. Empty the trash. Carry a sofa. There are heavy things on the ground that you need to pick up. It happens all day long, and there's no more functional movement in life, or in the gym, than this magnificent act. Best of all, whether you know it or not, you're deadlifting every time.

It's safe to assume the deadlift is the oldest strength-training maneuver in existence. There's no real documentation to back this up, but it makes perfect sense when you think about it. Benching and squatting took our forefathers some ingenuity to contrive, but picking something up? Putting it down and picking it up again? That's instinct.

A caveman points at a rock. He tells another to pick it up. If the guy can, he gets to eat a raw wooly mammoth steak. If he can't, he's clubbed over the head. Those were the stakes in the world's first powerlifting meet, and not much has changed since then. Deadlift training technique and programming have been refined, but the main objective remains the same: you pick things up and put them down. Here's how it's done.

Deadlifting for Strength

Ripping a heavy barbell off the floor requires a serious commitment. To get stronger, the idea is to develop the confidence to know a lift is complete before you even wrap your hands around the barbell, every time you deadlift. Come hell or high water, you have to keep pulling.

Though deadlifting seems ridiculously simple, the lift has several technical aspects you'll need to master to make progress. By learning to use your body's natural leverages and finding your "groove," you'll both lift heavier weights and prevent injuries.

Proper technique starts with your stance. To find yours, perform a standing vertical jump, noting the width of your feet at the start. This foot position, with your toes pointed out slightly, is your new deadlift stance. From here, descend into a half squat with the barbell — which sits over the centers of your feet — touching your shins and your arms fully extended.

Your workouts for this strength cycle are designed to develop two cornerstones of correct deadlifting technique. First, you'll be using compensatory acceleration training (CAT) every time you perform a deadlift. This means every rep will be done as fast and explosively as possible — even your warm-up sets. Next, with every rep, focus on pushing your heels through the ground while making sure your hips don't rise faster than your shoulders. Keeping your hips down will prevent your legs from locking out before your hips, a mistake that will take away significant amounts of power and leave your hamstrings and lower back vulnerable to injury.

The workout template provided is a six-week cycle designed to increase your deadlift max by as much as 10 percent. On day one, you'll deadlift. On day two, you'll perform a series of accessory squat variations with direct carryover to your deadlift strength.

Once your technical proficiency improves and you're adding more weight to the bar, you'll notice that deadlifting works virtually every muscle in your body, with an emphasis on the muscles of your posterior chain: your glutes, hamstrings and lower back. Working these muscle groups independently with your assistance exercises is crucial to developing the lower body strength you'll need for a powerful pull.

Shrugs, barbell rows and weighted chin-ups will add mass to your upper back and allow you to pull heavier weight to the standing, locked-out top position of the deadlift. Rows and chins also provide your workouts with balance by having you perform pulling movements in both the vertical and horizontal planes. For your glutes and hamstrings, there's no better movement than the glute-ham raise, a movement requiring a powerful co-contraction of these two massive muscle groups.

Deadlifting for Size

Ronnie Coleman has a big back. It's big enough for eight Mr. Olympia titles, big enough that calling it "big" qualifies as understatement, and big enough for you to pay close attention to how he built it. Brian Dobson, Coleman's longtime trainer, attributes Big Ron's massive back to one factor that's remained constant in his training programs through the years. "Deadlifts," says Dobson, "are the king."

Deadlifting forces you to use virtually every muscle in your body to take the bar from the floor to waist height. In the chain of muscles involved in this process, nothing is left behind and everything kicks in, eventually.

Everything starts with your lower back. Nothing builds your spinal erectors like the repetitive action of bearing and moving a massive load. The deadlift isn't just a lower back exercise, though. As you move through your range of motion and transition from the lower part of the lift to the upper lockout phase, your lats, traps and other upper-back muscles take over. At the top of the movement, you're holding a very heavy weight in a dead hang potion – which places immense pressure on your traps. This is a very efficient combination of movements for building thickness in your upper back and shoulders.

In the bottom position, proper deadlift technique entails pushing through your heels to move the bar out of a static position. By focusing on this leg drive, you're applying a tremendous amount of force to your quads, hamstrings and calves. Dropping your ass and pushing through your heels with every rep will add mass throughout your lower body.

At the top of the deadlift, when you lock out your hips, your glutes act as the movement's agonist — its prime mover — while your hamstrings are targeted as the synergists, or assisters. When it comes to developing your glutes and hamstrings through the application of force, there's no better exercise than the deadlift.

The benefits aren't limited to your lower body. Your arms come into play throughout your range of motion. When you're both trying to hang onto a heavy load and move it upward, all the muscles in your arms are forced to contract, in addition to the obvious necessity for grip and forearm strength and mass development.

The routine provided here targets muscular hypertrophy with reps in the 6-15 range, as opposed to our strength routine, which focuses more on heavier sets for lower reps. Research by Dr. Eric Serrano has shown the importance of prolonging the time muscles are under tension during a set. Keeping your time-under-tension between 30-60 seconds – especially in the deadlift, where so many muscle groups are in play – will elicit the greatest muscle-building response from your resistance training. Keep your rest periods at two minutes or less for your main exercises each day, and take full advantage of the incredible growth hormone response deadlifting can produce.

Important Notes to Remember:

1. Push through your heels.
2. The middle of your foot should be directly under the bar, with your shins touching the bar.
3. Extend your back. Don't round it.
4. Your shoulder blades should be over the bar, with your shoulders in front of it.
5. Pull with your hips, not with your arms.
6. Position your hands slightly outside your thighs.
7. Maintain full extension in your elbows throughout your range of motion.
8. Don't deadlift in front of a mirror. Even the slightest adjustment in form can cause serious injury.
9. Squeeze your glutes tightly to prevent pulling with your lower back.
10. Lower the bar exactly how your raised it.

8 Week Strength Building Deadlift Routine

The "Get Stronger" Deadlift Program				
Weeks 1-4				
Exercise	Sets/Reps	Sets/Reps	Sets/Reps	Sets/Reps
	Week 1	Week 2	Week 3	Week 4/Deload
Deadlift	1x3 (75%)	1x3 (80%)	1x3 (85%)	6x1 (60%)
Speed Deadlift	3x6 (60%; Rest 60 Sec.)	3x8 (60%; Rest 60 Sec.)	3x6 (70%; Rest 60 Sec.)	Off
3-Inch Deficit Deadlift	2x5 (65%)	2x5 (68%)	2x4 (75%)	Off
Bent Over Row	3x8	3x7	3x6	2x5 (60%)
Shrug	3x12	3x12	3x12	3x6 (70% of weight used on week 3)
Glute Ham Raise (or 45 degree Back)	3x8	3x8	3x8	2x6
The "Get Stronger" Deadlift Program				
Weeks 5-8				
Exercise	Sets/Reps	Sets/Reps	Sets/Reps	Sets/Reps
	Week 5	Week 6	Week 7/Deload	Week 8 MAX
Deadlift	1x2 (90%)	1x1 (95%)	6x1 (60%)	MAXOUT
Speed Deadlift	4x2 (75%; Rest 120 Sec.)	3x2 (80%; Rest 120 Sec.)	Off	
3-Inch Deficit Deadlift	3x3 (80%0	3x3 (82.5%)	Off	
DB Row	3x6	3x6	2x5 (60%)	
Shrug	3x10	3x10	3x6 (70% of weight used on week 6)	
Glute Ham Raise (or 45 degree Back)	3x8	3x7	2x6	

8 Week Size Building Deadlift Routine

The "Get Bigger" Deadlift Program				
Weeks 1-4				
Exercise	Sets/Reps	Sets/Reps	Sets/Reps	Sets/Reps
	Week 1	Week 2	Week 3	Week 4/Deload
Stiff Leg Deficit Deadlift	5x10 (30,35,40,45,35%)	5x10 (30,40,50,37.5%)	5x10 (30,40,47.5,52.5,40%)	3x10 (30%)
Shrug	4x25	4x25	4x25	2x20 (60%)
Bent Over Row	4x10	4x10	4x10	2x10 (60%)
Wide Pull Up	3x6	3x6	3x6	2x5
Narrow Pull Up	3x6	3x6	3x6	2x5
Incline Sit Up	3x15	3x15	3x15	3x15
The "Get Bigger" Deadlift Program				
Weeks 5-8				
Exercise	Sets/Reps	Sets/Reps	Sets/Reps	Sets/Reps
	Week 5	Week 6	Week 7	Week 8/Deload
Regular Deficit Deadlift	5x6 (45,50,55,60,50%)	5x6 (50,55,60,70,55%)	5x6 (50,55,65,75,60%)	3x6 (40%)
Shrug	4x15	4x15	4x15	2x15 (60%)
Bent Over Row	3x8	3x8	3x8	2x8 (60%)
Wide Pull Up	2x9	2x9	2x9	1x9
Narrow Pull Up	2x9	2x9	2x9	1x9
Incline Sit Up	3x15	3x15	3x15	3x15

Time to hit the pig iron!

V-Taper Back Workout

It takes the right combination of exercises to build a thick back, shoulders that flare, and a narrow waistline to pull off the best V-shaped symmetry. A lot of people make the mistake of focusing only on lifting heavy weight or doing a ton of reps, never paying attention to exactly how long their muscles are under continuous tension.

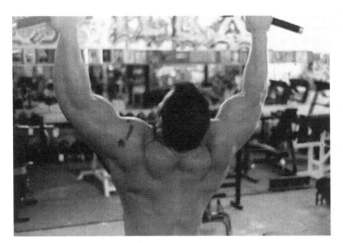

When you apply this high-intensity technique, however, your muscles spend more time contracted and activate more fibers than usual. This can help build more size in less time, especially if you're new to the technique.

Train back and shoulders only once a week with two to three days of rest in between sessions (that's two to three days of rest between Day 1 and Day 2 of the training program). Do not mix these workouts with anything else on the same day – the volume is too intense. Go by feel instead of the clock when it comes to rest intervals between sets. Allow yourself sufficient recovery time with the heavier compound exercises such as deadlifts, presses, and rows. Try running through the isolation movements at the quickest pace you can handle. We recommend at least two to three minutes of rest between sets of compound moves and 45-60 seconds between isolation exercises.

				V-Taper Back Workout

Day	Exercise	Sets	Reps	Comments
Day 1	Deadlift	4	10,8,6,12	Do pyramid-style reps, adding weight each set. If the reps increase on the last set, strip off some weight. Don't use earlier sets to warm up – each set should be difficult.
	Bent Over Row	5	12,12,10,8,6	Do pyramid-style reps, adding weight each set. If the reps increase on the last set, strip off some weight. Don't use earlier sets to warm up – each set should be difficult.
	Weighted "21" Pull Up	4	21	Start: Grasp an overhead bar with your hands just wider than your shoulders and have a partner place a 10 to 20-pound dumbbell between your legs just below your knees. Hang freely with your arms extended but elbows unlocked.Execute: Slowly pull yourself up until the bar is above your chest, return to the start and repeat for seven reps. Swap the dumbbell for one that is half as heavy, then do seven more reps. Finally, drop the weight and do seven bodyweight reps. Rest and repeat the 21-rep sequence, this time gripping the narrow parallel bars. Add weight as you get stronger. If you are not strong enough to do this move with weight, start with seven bodyweight pull-ups and gradually increase the amount of resistance using either a machine or a partner's help.
	Standing Low Cable Row	5	15	Attach a V-bar to a low-pulley cable. Stand facing the stack with your knees slightly bent, your feet wider than your shoulders and your back flat. Bend at the hips to grasp the attachment with both hands, arms extended.Slowly pull the handle towards your midsection, pause for a count, then slowly return the bar back to the start.
	Straight Arm Pulldown	5	12	Stand erect a few feet in front of a high-pulley cable, feet slightly wider than your hips for stability. Reach up and grasp the bar with an overhand grip, hands just outside shoulder width.Keeping your arms straight and your torso erect, slowly pull the bar down to your thighs. Slowly return to the start position.
	One Arm DB Row	5	10	Stand Alongside a flat bench with a dumbbell in your left hand. Place your right hand and knee on the bench, and lean forward at the hips until your back is almost parallel to the floor. Let your left arm hang straight toward the floor, palm facing in.Slowly pull the weight up to your side, pause, and return to the start. On the final rep, pause at the top for 10 seconds. Switch sides and repeat.
Day2	Partner Partial DB Press	3	90, 75,60 Sec.	Stand erect holding a pair of dumbbells overhead, elbows locked.When your partner yells "go," quickly lower the weights to your shoulders, then press them back up halfway. Repeat, then lower the weights and press them overhead with your elbows locked. Repeat this three-step movement (half rep, half rep, full rep) as fast as you can for time. Your partner should monitor your efforts so you reach failure by the end of each set. To keep your muscles guessing, vary your rest between cycles from 1-5 seconds.
	Standing DB Shrug	4	10	Stand erect with a heavy dumbbell in each hand, arms at your sides, and palms facing in. Raise your left shoulder as high as you can toward your ear and lower it back down, resisting the urge to bend your elbow. Repeat for reps, then switch sides. Finish the set by raising both shoulders simultaneously for reps.
	Around The Wrold	3	10,8,6	Stand erect holding a weight plate with both hands in front of your abs, arms just shy of full extension.Lift the plate overhead and circle it clockwise around your head for reps. Reverse the motion and circle the plate counterclockwise for reps. Finish the set by raising the plate overhead and lowering it to your thighs for reps.
	Lateral T-Raise	5	15,12,10,8,15	Stand erect with a dumbbell in each hand, upper arms pinned to your sides and your elbows bent 90 degrees. Your forearms should be parallel to the floor with your palms facing in.Raise your elbows out to your sides until your palms face down and your upper arms are parallel to the floor. Return to the start.
	Face Pulls	5	15	Stand erect in front of a lat pulldown station and grasp the bar with an overhand grip, hands wider than shoulder-width apart. For balance, place one foot on the seat and lean back so your body is at a 45-degree angle.Maintaining this position, retract your shoulders to pull the bar toward your face. Return slowly (resisting the weight as you go) until your arms are straight.

The prescribed workout will build the proportionate mass; we will shed body fat with HIIT. Any type of activity will do — cycling, running, skipping rope, shadowboxing, even hitting the heavy bag — as long as it does not affect your strength levels when you lift. We recommend using the rating of perceived exertion (RPE) scale to regulate the intensity of your intervals: rate how hard you are working on a scale of 1 (easy) to 10 (hard).

Weeks 1-2
30 minutes of high-intensity interval training, 2-3 days a week
Weeks 3-4
30 minutes of high-intensity interval training, 3-4 times a week
Weeks 5-6
30 minutes of high-intensity interval training, 3-4 times a week
Weeks 1-6
30-45 minutes of low-intensity activity (walking or hiking), 1-2 days a week
Time to hit the pig iron!

Back Training—Minimum Time, Maximum Results!

Ronnie Coleman, Lee Haney and Dorian Yates have the best three backs in the history of bodybuilding, and nearly half of the Sandows ever handed out since the Olympia's inception.

"Strong man equals strong back," said Bill Kazmaier, the strongest man to ever walk the earth. A man with a thick, wide back screams functional power and seeps with masculine virility.

Not everyone has hours a day to dedicate to back training. If you are willing to give your all once a week for 45 minutes, you can take your back development to a whole new level with the following routine.

Since the time is short, 100-percent concentration is needed in the gym.

Lack of time is no excuse for lack of results. We are going to dedicate ourselves to just three exercises.

Deadlifts

Ronnie Coleman, the most muscular, strongest bodybuilder of all-time, had heavy deadlifts at the core of his back routine. Johnny Jackson fills out doorjambs and terrorizes tailors with the best back in pro bodybuilding today, and officially deadlifted 832 raw under Josh's tutelage in 2012.

It is no coincidence that heavy deadlifts are synonymous with great back development.

Instead of deadlifting for hours on end, efficiency is the name of the game. After you are warmed up, you have 12 minutes to complete all deadlifts. Start with a weight you are capable of doing 8-10 reps with. For set one do five reps.

Rest 60 seconds and attempt five reps again; if you are unable to complete five reps do four, if you cannot do four reps do three, if you cannot do three reps do two, and if two reps is too much, do one. Always stop one shy of failure but do not exceed five repetitions. Repeat this process for 12 minutes. The clock starts once you have completed your first set.

On the last set, if you still have something left, go for an all-out rep max stopping one repetition shy of failure.

When you can complete 40 repetitions in this time period, increase the weight on the bar by five percent; if you cannot, make sure you beat your previous rep record.

No sumo deadlifts!

We want to build muscle and functional power.

Some reminders for proper deadlift technique:

- Push through your heels
- The middle of the foot should be directly under the bar
- Shins should touch the bar
- The back is in extension; don't round it
- The shoulder blades should be directly over the bar, and shoulders will be slightly in front
- The elbows must remain in full extension throughout the entire movement
- Lower the bar in the opposite way the bar was lifted in terms of hip and knee angles

Meadows Rows

This movement comes from bodybuilder John Meadows. It is like a one-armed dumbbell row, but uses a T-bar instead. Stand next to the end you would normally load plates on, grab the handle with one hand and row with it; it is important to wear straps because the end of the bar is fat and we are aiming for a back workout, not a grip test.

While rowing exercises have long been known for building thick backs, done correctly, this could be almost considered a "width" movement. Meadows recommends slightly kicking your hips away from the bar and emphasizing the stretch, which you will feel in the lower lats.

Instead of counting reps, pick a weight you can do 15 reps with. Start with your weakest arm by performing as many reps as possible in one minute, emphasizing stretch and technique; rest one minute and match this number of reps on the stronger arms. Rest one minute, then do the same thing for 45 seconds on the original arm; rest 45 seconds and follow suit on the weaker arm. Rest 45 seconds and the final set on the strong arm go for 30 seconds, rest 30 seconds and finish for 30 seconds on the weaker arm.

This will take a total of eight minutes and 30 seconds.

Straight-Arm Pull-Downs

Doug Young held the bench press world record for many years with a 611 RAW in the 275-pound weight class. Doug was the quintessential powerbuilder, having strength coupled with a symmetrical physique that irradiated power; in fact, Young served as a mass consultant to Arnold Schwarzenegger.

In every upper body workout, Young included six sets of straight-arm pull-downs. With a tapered waist and wide lats, Doug Young looked like a superhero.

In some pulling movements, the limiting factor is the biceps. Because they are involved and they fatigue before the back, straight-arm pull-downs are an isolation movement that work great for building back width and circumventing the limited biceps.

How to correctly perform a straight-arm pull-down:

- Grab a straight bar or rope attachment on a pulling machine
- Step backward about two feet facing the machine
- Fully extend your arms
- Bend your torso slightly forward
- Tighten your lats
- Pull the bar down using your lats until your hands are down to your thighs
- Make sure you keep this movement strict; if you start to cheat, it becomes ineffective
- Return to starting position, always staying under control

We are going to do this movement for two minutes straight! Pick a weight you can do 15-20 reps with. You are going to do three reps, slow and controlled, and after the three reps are complete, hold the weight in the top position emphasizing the stretch for five seconds. Repeat the process and do this for two minutes.

Huge Back Routine				
Exercise	Sets	Reps	Intensity	Rest Interval
Deadlift	MAX	1--5	8-10RM	60 Sec.
Meadows Rows	3	MAX	15RM	60,45,30 Sec.
Straight Arm Pulldowns	MAX	3	15--20	See Description

Final Thoughts

There's nothing cute and nothing fancy about this workout. This is the bare-bone basics! It's time to build a back that fills out doorjambs and terrorizes tailors.

Time to hit the pig iron!

Partial Training for Full Development

Full range of motion for full development is generally a good rule of thumb, but like the old proverb says, there is a time and a place for everything.

Partial reps are a movement performed in a specific range of motion. For the bench press, an example would be a board press; for the deadlift, a rack pull; and for the military press, a press to the top of the head.

Partial reps allow for an overload. In other words, you can use more weight in a partial range of motion than a full range of motion, which will help your central nervous system adapt to heavier weights, along with providing a huge psychological boost as you climb the intensity ladder of heavy weights. After all, how intimidating is 300-pound bench press if you have done a 405-pound bench press off of four boards?

Partials can additionally work specific range of motion, i.e., attacking sticking points.

Let's use the bench press as an example.

If you have a sticking point at the four-board height, your training weights could potentially be held back. By overloading that sticking point and eliminating it, you can now handle heavier weights on a full-range-of-motion bench press, which means fully developed pecs. Additionally, by handling supramaximal weights, you will also strengthen connective tissue.

Remember, while partial reps are great for handling heavier weights, you should also work them at your weakest points. Many times, this might mean using less weight than you could perform through a full range of motion. That's because you're in your individual worst leverage point, but this will ultimately help you blow past your sticking point and eventually handle more weight throughout the full range of motion.

Partial-rep training guidelines:

- Partials are very demanding and, if overdone, can induce central and peripheral fatigue because you are lifting beyond your one-rep max. Do not do partials more than three weeks in a row without a deload (period of lower intensity).
- Keep full-range-of-motion movements in your program; do not use exclusively partials or include partials every single session. Ultimately, our base training is a full range of motion, and we do not want to adversely affect neurological adaptations to full-range-of-motion movements. In other words, if you do too many partials, your full-range-of-motion movements will feel extremely awkward.
- Use periodization training with partial movements. Do not perform partials more than three weeks in a row without a deload. After the deload, one more 3-week mesocycle can be completed, and then you can take time off from partials.
- Overload and work weak points.
- Make sure you are mentally and physically prepared for partial reps. You have to make sure you are tight; you are lifting more than your max!

Partial Back Workout		
Exercise	Sets	Reps
Rack Pull-18 Inches	3	3
Rack Pull Overload-8 Inch ROM	3	5
Deadlift	3	6
Chin Up RP	1	(3 Rest Pauses)
Wide Grip Lat Pulldown	3	12
Meadows Rows	3	8

If you train only with partials, you will experience only partial development. Correct implementation of partials can be an integral part of building a championship physique.

Time to hit the pig iron!

8-Week Neck Blast

In generations past, any serious strength-training regimen included neck work. As things "advanced" (or self-castrated), finding a lifter doing neck work was as likely as Liberace performing at a Jerry Falwell rally.

Is it any wonder that study after study shows men's testosterone levels plummeting?

A muscular, well-developed neck is synonymous with power, and its mere existence commands a certain level of respect from fellow humans. Whether you are a bouncer at the famed Kentucky Club in Juarez, Mexico, or a CEO leading a Fortune 500 company, having a burly neck sends off a "don't screw with me" message.

Baggy shirts cover up lack of upper body development and baggy pants hide the fact you repeatedly skipped leg day (think Justin Bieber), but there is no garment that can hide your "stack of dimes," pencil neck!

Some of us iron game "old heads" won't let neck work die this easily. I am inviting you to join us in our quest to preach the gospel of the importance of a strong neck!

Powerful-Neck Epiphany

When I was a junior in high school, my best friend, Adam benShea, and I really wanted to go to a bar after watching the movie Roadhouse for the umpteenth time.

Being in Southern California, Mexican bars were a dime a dozen, especially in Oxnard. One day we decided to make the 45-minute journey and head down to the "Nard." We ended up at this little Mexican kick-and-stab called the Roadhouse (yes, the name influenced us).

Much to our astonishment, we saw a familiar face at this Mexican joint. At the time, we had been working out at the Gold's Gym in Oxnard with our lifting mentor, Steve Holl, and at the Roadhouse was a wannabe bodybuilder from that gym. He was the typical all-show-no-go, "pec and bi warrior." Suddenly, some sort of argument erupted between the wannabe bodybuilder and a few other patrons. Next thing we knew, a simian-like bouncer rushed out of the back sporting traps like a silver back gorilla. He had one of the thickest, most imposing necks I had ever seen. The sequoia-like neck on this man was something that will forever be etched in my memory. It was like a scene out of a movie; everything came to a screeching halt when this behemoth came rushing out of the back… it fell silent and the girls on stage stopped dancing and stared intently at the situation unfolding.

The bouncer walked toward the puffed-up pretty boy and proceeded to put his hands behind his own back, approaching the bodybuilder in a passive stance. The bouncer walked right up to the "bodybuilder's" face and told him to leave immediately (followed up with some words that would have sailors blushing).

The pretty boy could have easily taken a cheap shot while the bouncer's hands were behind his back, but he knew better. The bouncer demonstrated power from a vulnerable position; it was very impressive to watch. To this day, it is one of the finest pieces of "bouncering" I have ever seen.

Adam looked at me and said, "It's the neck." He didn't have to say it; I knew it was the reason the bouncer was able to command the room. That was the day I realized the power of a strong, muscular neck. I made a promise to myself that I would never neglect my own neck training.

Functional Benefits of a Strong Neck

"When a warrior goes to battle, he must have a sword and a shield. The neck is the fighter's shield." – Adam benShea, former Brazilian Jiu-Jitsu World Champion

A strong, muscular neck will reduce a fighter's chance of getting knocked out or choked out. In fact, having a strong neck will reduce the likelihood of neck or head injuries during any physical collision, whether it is in an automobile or on the football field.

Football "sports performance specialists" that do ladder drills 'til the cows come home but neglect neck work should be publicly pistol-whipped or banished to Planet Fitness.

Big Lifts = Big Neck?

Compound movements are the most efficient movements and need to be at the core of any program geared toward strength, size, or fat loss.

But some believe that performing just a few big lifts will equal big gains all over. While it is true that the average serious weight-trainer has a more-developed neck than the average Joe on the street, to maximize neck strength and size, you have to directly train your neck.

The *European Journal of Applied Physiology and Occupational Physiology* confirmed this from a landmark study published in 1997 entitled, "Specificity of resistance training responses in neck muscle size and strength."

The study consisted of three groups. First was a resistance-training group that trained performing squats, deadlifts, push presses, high pulls and barbell rows. The second resistance-training group performed the same strength-training movements in addition to neck extensions with a harness three times a week. The third group did not workout at all.

The resistance-training group that did not train neck extensions did not increase neck strength. Contrast this with the subjects that performed neck-extension work, they increased neck-extension strength by a staggering 34 percent over the 12-week duration of the study. Also, the group that performed neck work increased the cross-sectional area of neck musculature by 13 percent compared to no increase for subjects that did not directly work the neck.

Bottom line: if you want a big, strong neck... you have to train your neck!

How Quickly Can This Happen?

The Naval Health Research Center demonstrated in a 2006 published study that significant increases in neck strength were evident in both static and dynamic strength assessments with a month of neck-resistance training. Total neck size increased by 13 percent, which can be the difference between an average neck and one that projects an aura of supremacy.

The study also showed that military personnel who regularly trained the neck had fewer injuries and far fewer sick days. We'd venture to say the same would hold true for the linebacker, the clergymen, or the Irish-gypsy bareknuckle prize-fighter.

So, we now know, according to the scientific literature, that significant increases in neck strength and size can be realized in as little as one to three months. But what is the best way to get a neck that will scare the gorillas at the zoo and command respect from your friends and foes at the back-alley poker game?

How Do I Train My Neck?

For help with this routine, we consulted a good friend, Texas Powerlifting legend Jim Voronin. At 380 pounds, Jim measured a 25.5-inch neck!

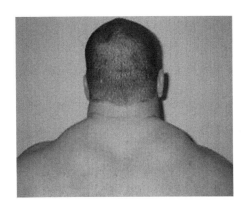

Jim was arguably the most dominant super heavy weight power-lifter of the 1990s, having dazzled crowds with his amazing size and strength from Juarez, Mexico, to Paris, France. Jim was also a successful strongman competitor. Today, Jim is a Powerlifting referee and Vice Principal. Jim gives back to the sport more than anyone.

Together, we put together this collar-busting neck routine.

On Day 2, for the isometric neck flexions, push your head downward against an immovable resistance for 10 seconds (if you have a four-way neck machine that is okay to substitute flexion for three sets of 10-15).

		8 Week Neck Blitz			
		Weeks 1-4			
Day	Exercise	Sets/Reps	Sets/Reps	Sets/Reps	Sets/Reps
		Week 1	Week 2	Week 3	Week 4
Day 1	Neck Harness	4x10	4x10	4x9	4x9
	Barbell Shrugs	2x20	2x20	2x20	2x20
	Barbell Shrugs	1x15-40	1x15-40	1x15-40	1x15-40
Day 2	Neck Harness	3x20	3x20	3x20	3x20
	Overhead Shrugs	3x15	3x15	3x15	3x15
	One Arm Barbell Shrugs	3x12	3x12	3x15	3x15
	Lateral Flexion	3x15	3x15	3x12	3x12
	Neck Flexion Isometrics	6x1	6x1	6x1	6x1
		8 Week Plan			
		Weeks 5-8			
Day	Exercise	Sets/Reps	Sets/Reps	Sets/Reps	Sets/Reps
		Week 5	Week 6	Week 7	Week 8
Day 1	Neck Harness	4x8	4x7	4x5	4x6
	Barbell Shrugs	2x20	2x20	2x20	2x20
	Barbell Shrugs	1x15-40	1x15-40	1x15-40	1x15-40
Day 2	Neck Harness	3x20	3x20	3x20	3x20
	Overhead Shrugs	3x15	3x12	3x12	3x12
	One Arm Barbell Shrugs	3x15	3x10	3x10	3x10
	Lateral Flexion	3x12	3x12	3x12	3x12
	Neck Flexion Isometrics	6x1	6x1	6x1	6x1

Guidelines

- Use a full range of motion (should this be smaller font)
- Go as heavy as possible without sacrificing form
- Progressively add weight
- Use rest Intervals of one to two minutes

Final Thoughts

Ask not what your neck can do you for you, but what you can do for your neck.

Let's build a neck that decreases your chance of real-life injury and radiates an aura of power that garners respect anywhere from Penn State to the state pen!

Time to hit the pig iron!

UPPER BODY

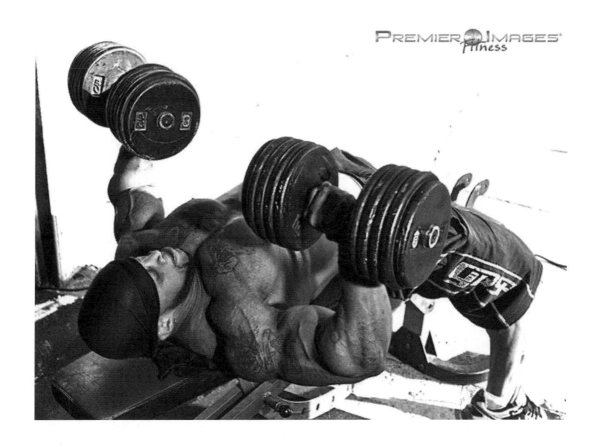

Power Rack Chest Training

So, your last heavy barbell pressing session coincided with a popular new dance at the time, "el Macarena."

Is it any wonder that your chest development resembles Macaulay Culkin's?

The issue may be a lack of spotters or training partners, but we have a solution!

Pushing sets to repetition maximums, partial overloads and virtually any strength-building barbell movement can be accomplished in solitude in the power rack!

Fail with a weight? No big deal, the pins, your "built in spotters," will allow you to flee to safety.

Here is the bottom line:

Go to the gym, park your ass in the power rack and do not leave until the workout is complete. This may not be the best way to win friends and influence people, but we are going to move away from Carnegie tradition and adopt the attitude of warlord Attila the Hun.

Remember, you are at the gym to train, not socialize. View everyone else as a silhouette.

Power Rack Chest Training Program			
Exercise	**Sets**	**Reps**	**Comment**
Bench Press	2	RP	Bench Presses have played an important role of virtually all iron game athletes that possess a big beautiful hood and strength to match. Full range of motion is the name game; make sure every bench press touches your chest, do not bounce reps. Sets are performed in a rest-pause style meaning, start with a weight you can perform for 5 to 8 repetitions with. Lift the weight for as many reps as possible, take a 20-second rest interval, and do the same weight again; this will probably be 2-3 repetitions.
Dead Bench	6	1	
Feet Elevated Push-Ups	1	Failure	
Reverse Grip Push-Ups	3	6,6,max	
Isometric Squeeze	6	10	

Take a three to four-minute rest interval between rest-pause sets.

Final Thoughts

If you have a power rack, a barbell, and weights you have no excuse not to have a great physique and strength levels to match.

Time to hit the pig iron!

8 Week Overhead Pressing Party

This routine will build masculine brawn, enhance utilitarian strength, and fulfill the traditional look of raw power. So, to build shoulders that take out doorjambs, fill out prison denim, and impress even the most jaded tailor, complete the following routine.

All exercises go as heavy as possible while maintaining good form, including adding weights to dips and pull-ups. Increase poundages weekly!

Day	Exercise	Sets/Reps	Sets/Reps	Sets/Reps	Sets/Reps
Raw Overhead Power					
Weeks 1-4					
		Week 1	Week 2	Week 3	Week 4/Deload
Day 1	Overhead Press	10x1 (75%; Rest 30 Sec.)	8x1 (80%; Rest 45 Sec.)	6x1 (83%; Rest 60 Sec.)	4x1 (60%)
	Bottom Level Isometric Followed By CAT OHP	(5 Second Push-Rest 2 Min-CAT OHPx3)X6	(5 Second Push-Rest 2 Min-CAT @ 65% OHPx1)X2	(5 Second Push-Rest 2 Min-CAT @ 65% OHPx1)X2	Off
	Mid Level Isometric Followed By CAT OHP	(5 Second Push-Rest 2 Min-CAT @ 65% OHPx1)X2	(5 Second Push-Rest 2 Min-CAT @ 65% OHPx1)X2	(5 Second Push-Rest 2 Min-CAT @ 65% OHPx1)X2	Off
	Top Level Isometric Followed By CAT OHP	(5 Second Push-Rest 2 Min-CAT @ 65% OHPx1)X2	(5 Second Push-Rest 2 Min-CAT @ 65% OHPx1)X2	(5 Second Push-Rest 2 Min-CAT @ 65% OHPx1)X2	Off
	Dips	3X8 (Heavy as Possible)	3x8 (Heavy as Possible)	3x7 (Heavy as Possible)	3x6 (70% of weight used on week 3)
	Neutral Grip Pull Ups	Juarez Valley 6 (6, 1, 5,2, 4, 3)	Juarez Valley 6	Juarez Valley 6 (As Heavy As Possible)	2x8 (70% of weight used on week 3)
	Standing Weighted Crunches	3x10	3x12	3x12	2x8 (70% of weight used on week 3)
Day 2	1-Arm Neutral DB Press	2xRest Pause (RP=Do as many as possible one shy of failure-rest 20 sec.-do another set one shy of failure-rest 20 sec.-repeat one last set=One set of RP)(Use 8RM weight and do weker arm first, then match reps on strong arm)	2xRP (@8RM)	2xRP (@5RM)	3x8 (60%; Rest 60 Sec.)
	Face Pulls	3x12	3x12	3x12	2x12 (60%)
	Lat Pull-Downs	3x10	3x10	3x8	2x8 (60%)
	Incline Chest Supported DB Rows	3x12	3x10	3x6	2x6 (60%)
	Overhead Dicks Press	5x8	5x8	5x8	3x8 (60%; Rest 60 Sec.)
	Cheat Curls	3x6 (5 Sec. Negative)	3x6 (5 Sec. Negative)	3x5 (5 Sec. Negative)	2x5

		Sets/Reps	Sets/Reps	Sets/Reps	Sets/Reps
Raw Overhead Power					
Weeks 5-8					
Day	Exercise	Week 5	Week 6	Week 7	Week 8/Deload
Day 1	OHP	5x1 Last Set RP (88%; Rest 90 Sec.)	92%x1 (Do as many sets as possible with 25 Sec. rest between)	96%x1 (Do as many sets as possible with 35 Sec. rest between)	3x3 (65%; Rest 60 Sec.)
	Land Mine Press	3x8	3x7	3x5	3x3 (55%)
	Dips	3x6	3x5	3x5	2x5
	Neutral Grip Pull Ups	Juarez Valley 6 (6,1,5,2,4,3)	Jailhouse 7 (7,6,5,4,3,2,1)	Jailhouse 7	3x5
	Overhead Tricep Extension 1-Arm DB	4x15	4x12	4x10	3x8 (60%; Rest 60 Sec.)
Day 2	Savickas Press	3x8	3x6	3x4	3x3 (65%; Rest 60 Sec.)
	Face Pulls	3x12	3x12	3x12	2x12 (60%)
	Lat Pull-Downs	3x8	3x8	3x8	3x6 (60%; Rest 60 Sec.)
	Incline Chest Supported DB Rows	3x8	3x7	3x8	3x5 (55%; Rest 60 Sec.)
	Overhead Dicks Press	5x6	5x5	5x5	2x5 (70% of weight used on weeks 7)
	Zottman Curls	3x15	3x12	3x10	2x10(70% of weight used on week 7)
Week 9 - MAXOUT					

Time to hit the pig iron!

■ ■ ■

Little Time, Big Chest

Everyone above ground is given 24 hours a day.

A majority of healthy, hard-training athletes sleep an average eight hours day. The average work day is now approaching nine hours, according to the Bureau of Labor Statistics.

Well, 17 hours of the day is gone. What about family and household responsibilities? As the responsibilities pile up, the available hours dwindle down. Unfortunately, the 24 hours in a day are nonnegotiable.

Oh yeah, that commute.

With that in mind, We are going to give you a workout that will take you no more than 30 minutes and will make your chesticles feel like they are going to explode.

This is going to be accomplished with giant sets; many abbreviated workout advocates avoid giant sets, like a deadly disease.

Why?

Giant sets are typically associated with 70s marathon bodybuilding workouts. This association is not false, but certainly taken out of context; giant set workouts don't need to take two to three hours.

Giant Sets — What and Why?

A giant set is four or more exercises paired together with minimal rest that target one body part. Done intensely enough, it will even provide cardiovascular benefits. Giant sets cause a spike in production of growth hormone and IGF-1. Giant sets are set up to target the trained muscle at various angles.

Giant sets increase metabolic stress because of the continuous sequence. Because the muscle is hit so hard and at so many different angles, exercise-induced muscle damage results, a key element in becoming large and in charge.

Broad-Shouldered Street Swoldier — Bill Pearl Style

Broad, developed shoulders add more to a physique than any other piece of anatomy.

In recent times, emaciated men have come to dominate the tinsel town flicks, but even toddlers have a tough time taking these action stars seriously. Classic-era action stars from John Wayne to Steve Reeves had one thing in common, broad shoulders!

As primordial as it sounds, the fact remains that wide shoulders inspire men and cause women to go wild.

Having powerfully-developed shoulders goes far beyond aesthetic appeal. The lumberjack or the prize fighter can significantly increase performance with strong, developed shoulders.

Shoulder development was the gold standard during the golden age of bodybuilding. What better place to look for guidance than to Bill Pearl? Pearl's bodybuilding championships spanned across three decades. Furthermore, he had a lot of go behind his show, regularly performing world-class feats of strength for his fans in exhibitions. Pearl accomplished all this while being a full-time gym owner and manufacturing weightlifting paraphernalia.

If your objective is to dominate prison-yard politics, fill out your clergy collar, or sports performance — well-developed shoulders are a necessity.

Bill Pearl Street Swoldier Routine			
Exercise	Sets	Reps	Comment
Wide Grip Upright Row	3	8	Compared to the narrow grip upright row, the wide grip is friendlier to the shoulder joint. Furthermore, contrasted to the narrow grip, the wide grip upright row variation was shown in a University of Memphis study recently to increase side delt activity and decrease biceps involvement. (McAllister et, al 2013.) Pearl, in the trenches, beat the lab to the punch by over half a century.
Seated Behind the Neck Press	4	8	In recent times, this movement has come under harsh scrutiny because of the risk to benefit ratio. If you have any shoulder issues, lack mobility or are apprehensive, substitute seated dumbbell shoulder presses. Be careful and emphasize technique.
Crucifix	3	8	This is an exercise seldom mentioned in the modern era, let's defer to the wisdom of Bill Pearl.
Seated Alternate Dumbbell Raise	3	8	This is basically a front raise on steroids.
Incline One Arm Lateral Raise	2	10	

Pearls of Wisdom

Wide-Grip Upright Row

Bill Pearl offers this advice: "This is a more difficult type of upright rowing exercise. The deltoids are worked more and much concentration is required to perform it correctly. Start with the barbell at arms' length, resting on the thighs, but with a wider than shoulder-width hand-spacing. Pull barbell up to a position at or above the nipples. Pause while contracting strongly, then lower to starting position. Inhale up, exhale down."

Go as heavy as possible each set, stopping one rep shy of momentary muscular failure. Take a rest of 90-120 seconds between sets.

Seated Behind-the-Neck Press

Interestingly, in EMG studies performed by Bret Contreras on a series of shoulder exercises for activities of all three deltoid heads and the traps, seated behind-the-neck presses vastly outshined other shoulder pressing variations for muscle activity.

Bill Pearl offers this advice: "This is performed as the regular standing press behind neck, only in a seated position. Rest the bar on your shoulders between each rep, and set yourself for the press."

Go as heavy as possible each set, stopping one rep shy of momentary muscular failure. Take a two- to three-minute rest between sets.

Crucifix

Pearl said that "To handle substantial poundage, stand in a solid position and press two dumbbells to arms' length overhead. Slowly lower them with straight arms and locked elbows to the sides at shoulder height. Attempt to hold arms in position for a count of five to 10. The purpose of the crucifix is to use the deltoids as a support and this places a stress of a different nature upon the muscles. Inhale while pressing the dumbbells overhead and exhale as they are lowered."

Go as heavy as possible each set, stopping one rep shy of momentary muscular failure. Take a rest of 60 seconds between sets.

Seated Alternate DB Raise

Pearl said: "Start with dumbbells held at arms' length at sides. With dumbbell in left hand in down position, raise dumbbell in right hand to arm's length overhead. Lower right arm to position hanging straight at side, raise the left arm. Inhale upward and exhale when lowering dumbbell."

Go as heavy as possible each set, stopping one rep shy of momentary muscular failure. Take a rest of 60 seconds between sets.

Final Words

If eight-minute abs is your thing, this probably isn't the routine for you. In the weight room, if you wear the proverbial blue collar, it's time to let the nuts hang and get to work.

Perform this routine once a week, twice if shoulders are lagging and up to three times for specialization. Enough chit chat — time to hit the pig iron!

Jailhouse Angled Chest Training

On the jailhouse weight pile, with limited equipment, inmates produce phenomenal gains. Because of a lack of equipment and crowded quarters, the con has two options: get creative and grow, or enter a muscle- and strength-building stalemate and risk getting punked in the shower.

My junior year in high school, I trained chest with two huge ex-cons who chose option A and taught me about Mechanical Advantage Drop sets and their necessity behind bars because of limited weights on the yard.

Limited weights at rush hour are a reality at most commercial gyms.

The Workout

After a few compound barbell-pressing exercises with very heavy weight, it was time for dumbbell incline presses. The bigger of the two muscled-up specimens barked at me to help him as he grabbed the 140s, sat back on a steep incline and proceeded to lift the dumbbells to failure — approximately eight reps.

Next, he sat up and said to drop the seat a couple holes and then hit five more reps. We then dropped the incline and he continued. As he reached failure, leverage (mechanical advantage) was improved by reducing the incline angle instead of by using less weight like traditional drop sets.

Drop Sets: Cheating?

Typically, a drop set consists of a total of two to three subsets and sets are typically reduced 10-30 percent per drop. Let's take a look at lateral raise. With strict form upon momentary muscular failure, slight "Body English" to overcome a sticking point can allow the set to continue.

Like a drop set, you continue by "cheating." Reducing the weight does not allow the set to continue. The set continues by lifting the weight in a stronger position.

Like "cheating," mechanical drop sets are simply lifting the weight in a stronger position upon failure, BUT unlike cheating, strict form can be kept.

Rest-Pause Training

Rest-pausing is when one can no longer continue and stops for a short period of time before continuing with the same weight. Like rest-pausing, one does not drop the weight with a mechanical advantage drop. In some instances, the weight does not have to be racked between drops, it may just be a change of stance or hand placement.

An example in the bench press is going from a narrow grip, to a wide grip, to your strongest grip.

			Mechanical Advantage Drop Set Routine		

Exercise	Sets	Reps	Comment
DB Incline Press	3	8,8,MADSx3	Set the adjustable incline bench to 45 degrees; pick a weight you can complete for ten repetitions. Complete two sets of 8 reps, on the final set take the weight to failure. Upon failure immediately lower the incline bench to 25 degrees and press the dumbbells to failure at this position, at failure lower the bench to a flat position and press the dumbbells to failure. Take a 3 minute rest interval between sets.
Narrow Grip Bench Press	3	8,8,MADSx3	On a flat bench perform two sets of 8 reps with a grip 6 inches closer than your strongest grip; pick a weight you can complete 10 repetitions with. On the third and final set press the weight to failure. Upon failure, rack the barbell take a grip 3 inches wider and press the weight to failure. Upon failure rack the barbell and take your strongest grip and press the weight to failure. Take a 3 minute rest interval between sets.
Incline DB Fly	3	12,12,MADSx3	Set the incline to 30 degrees and perform 12 dumbbell flys for 2 sets with a weight you are capable of performing 15 repetitions with. On the final set perform the flys to failure, upon failure lower the adjustable bench to a flat position and perform flys to failure, upon failure in the flat position without dropping the weight press the dumbbells with a neutral grip to failure. Take a 90 second rest interval between sets.
Push Up	1	MADSx1	Perform push-ups with feet elevated on a bench to failure; upon failure immediately perform push-ups on the floor to failure, immediately after failure on the floor get on your knees in a "girl push-up" position and perform push-ups on the knees to failure.
Isometric Poses	1	8	To finish off the workout grasp your palms together squeeze as hard as possible flexing your chest for ten seconds, do this 8 times. Take a 10 second rest between maximal isometric contractions.

Final Thoughts

Mechanical drop sets are equally as effective for the guy doing a 12-year stint behind bars as the guy doing a daily 12-hour stint in an office cubicle.

More weight on the bar, with more time under tension, and better form, equals superior results.

Time to hit the pig iron!

The Ultimate Dumbbell Routine

In days of yore, gyms catered to folks with serious strength and physique goals. Barbells, dumbbells and lifting platforms were the norm and the catalyst for building massive, powerful men.

Nowadays, some popular chain gyms have pizza night, alarms that go off from dropping weights, and floors filled with chrome machines.

This has caused a revolt, and many serious trainees are setting up home gyms. These "garage gorillas" and "cellar dwellers" (in the words of Brooks Kubik) are making great gains and finding their pig-iron nirvana.

Many home gyms are seriously limited on space and only have room for dumbbells; with adjustable dumbbells or power blocks, literally one set of handles is all that is needed.

The travelling salesman may work 16-hour days on the road. His training may be limited to a hotel gym and hotel gyms are limited with dumbbells.

With nothing more than a pair of dumbbells and a burning desire, you can build world-class strength and a world-class physique.

Give the following workout a shot.

If you are not familiar with tempo training, here is a brief synopsis:

The first number '3' is the time in seconds to lower the weight after you've reached the top of the lift. This is the eccentric, or negative, phase.

The second number '0' is the pause at the completion of the exercise or at the start of the lift.

The third character 'X' means an explosive lift in the concentric phase. This could be the lifting of the dumbbell in an arm curl in the concentric phase, for example. X just stands for explosive movement.

The fourth number '1' is the pause at the top of the lift, or when you have bent the elbow and lifted the dumbbell to the highest point in an arm curl.

Day	Exercise	Sets/Reps	Tempo
DB Training Routine			
Day 1	1a) Chest Supported DB Row	5x12	3111
	1b) Reverse Grip DB Bench Press	5x8	3111
	2a) DB Row to Hip	3x6 Each Sice	5111
	2b) DB Incline Bench Press	3x10	5111
	3a) DB Pullover	3x12	3121
	3b) DB Fly	3x8	3121
Day2	1a) DB Bulgarian Split Squat	3x8	3111
	1b) Zottman Curls	3x10	3111
	DB Keystone Deadlift	4	3111
	3a) DB Reverse Lunge	3x10	
	3b) Incline DB Curls	3x10	3111
	Standing DB Calf Raise	3x15	
Day3	1a) DB Military Press	3x6	3111
	1b) DB Shrugs	3x12	
	2a) Incline Lateral Raise	3x8	5111
	2b) DB Decline Tricep Extension	3x12	3111
	3a) DB Inverted Fly	3x15	3111
	3b) Tate Press	3x20	

Time to hit the pig iron!

The Ticket to the Gun Show

"Circumstances…what are circumstances? I make circumstances."
— Napoleon

Wipe away your crocodile tears if those strings of spaghetti that hang from your sleeves have not grown since the Bush administration left office.

We are going to create circumstances that will set free even the harshest prisoners of poor arm genetics. If you have the work ethic — we've got the plan!

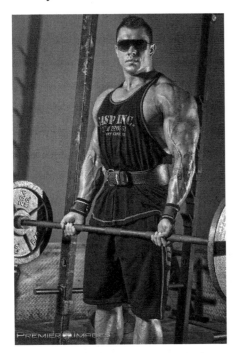

Far too many folks drink the Kool Aid of all that matters is "the pump" when training arms, pumping out set after set using very high reps with pygmy weights. Science confirms the pump does contribute to muscle growth, BUT mechanical tension (a.k.a., lifting heavy-ass pig iron) is the most important factor.

Important Notes: Dips, declines and skull-crushers are performed in a giant-set fashion. Move from one exercise to the next as quickly as possible. You will perform a total of three giant sets with a rest interval of five minutes between giant sets. Using a heavy, low-rep set, a moderate set in the traditional hypertrophy, and a very high-rep set, is a concept borrowed from, Fred Hatfield, which has served our clients very well.

The purpose of the giant set is to tax as many motor units as possible, from the High Threshold Motor Units to the small ones. Maximum muscular development requires a holistic approach; that's why we use a wide variety of rep ranges, time under tension and intensity levels.

Gun Show Workout 1

Exercise	Sets/Reps	Comments
Dips	3x5	Besides the anecdotes, dips were one of the few exercises that provided significant overload to all three heads of the triceps as demonstrated by MRI scans in Per Tesch's epic classic Targeted Bodybuilding. Because triceps make up 2/3 of the upper arm—we will start with what's most important first. We will commence with dips.
Decline Skull Crushers	3x10	Like dips, this was one of the few exercises that provided significant overload to all three heads of the triceps as demonstrated by MRI scans in Per Tesch's epic classic *Targeted Bodybuilding*.
Overhead Rope Extension	3x40	Using a slow, rhythmic style, the set should take at least 60 seconds to complete, ideally between 90 seconds and two minutes; do not stop, keep continuous tension on the triceps. Make sure you get a good stretch each rep
Hercules Chin Up	2x6	The Hercules chin-up is a creation of the Jailhouse Strong training system that uses incremental movements to build Herculean biceps. Pull yourself up until your chin is over the bar and hold for two seconds. Then, descend halfway down and hold for two seconds. Then repeat this movement for the prescribed number of repetitions. Finish with arms fully extended at the bottom. Add weight if possible; go as heavy as possible each set. Between sets take a two-minute rest interval. Make sure chin is completely over the bar and focus intentionally on the bicep contraction.
Narrow Grip Barbell Curls	2x15	Taking a narrow grip, with hands spaced approximately 6 to 8 inches apart, perform strict, full range of motion barbell curls as heavy as possible. Use a straight bar because this keeps your hands supinated (underhand grip) throughout the entirety of the movement, supination is a function of the biceps. Furthermore, a narrow grip puts all of the elbow flexors under extreme duress, a good thing for building the prize show guns.
Towel Hangs	20 Sec. 2x1	Muscled-up forearms ooze out an aura of power and scream don't screw with me! Having a grip like a vice is helpful in beer room brawling, on the field of play, or meeting your future father-in-law for the first time. Drape a towel over a pull-up bar and hang from the towel for 20 seconds, this should be difficult, if it is not, add weight. Heavy is the objective!

Important Notes: One-armed eccentric barbell curls, Gironda perfect curls and incline dumbbell curls are performed in a giant-set fashion. Move from one exercise to the next as quickly as possible. You will perform a total of three giant sets with a rest interval of five minutes between giant sets.

Exercise	Sets/Reps	Comments
One Armed Eccentric Barbell Curls	*3x5*	Numerous studies show that eccentric/negative contractions are a catalyst for muscle growth. Instead of just slowing down the negative, to truly maximize muscularity, you have to train eccentric emphasis movements. Eccentrics allow for preferential fast-twitch muscle fiber recruitment (a.k.a., the largest muscle fibers with the most potential for growth), prolonged time under tension, and much heavier loads can be used. Sit or stand behind a preacher curl station. Rest your upper arm on the pad in front of you, arms supinated. Start at the top position of the curl. Slowly lower the bar for a count of eight seconds to full extension. Pause briefly at the bottom. If you have a training partner, have him help you back up. If not, self-spot with the other hand.
Gironda Perfect Curls	*3x10*	This is not a cheat curl; there should be no swinging of the torso. The concentric should stake three seconds, the eccentric four seconds and hold the top position for one second. It almost feels like doing a heavy overload barbell curl with an incline stretch curl. Use a straight bar or EZ curl bar. Before starting the curls, bring your upper torso backward (shifting your weight toward the heels). The shoulders are now aligned behind the hips and knees in the starting position in a "stretched position." From this position, slowly curl the weight; as you lift the weight slowly bend the torso forward so at the end of the movement the shoulders are in front of the knees and the hips. I envision a giant "crunch" movement building a perfect bicep peak. Lower in the opposite motion back to the starting position.
Incline DB Curls	*3x40*	Sit or stand behind a preacher curl station. Rest your upper arm on the pad in front of you, arms supinated. Start at the top position of the curl. Slowly lower the bar for a count of eight seconds to full extension. Pause briefly at the bottom. If you have a training partner, have him help you back up. If not, self-spot with the other hand.
Close Grip Bench Press	*2x6*	With a shoulder width or narrow grip, use 75 percent of your strongest grip bench press maximum and perform your maximum number of reps. Repeat the process next with 65 percent of your max; finally finish your last set with 55 percent of your maximum lift.
Four Way Forearm	*2x15*	We will do four separate movements consecutively with a dumbbell, moving from movement to movement as fast possible without setting down the dumbbell. Each movement will be performed for 10 repetitions

Gun Show Workout 2

Four-Way Forearm

Movement 1 - With the wrist, move the dumbbell toward the midline of the body; moving the little finger side of the hand toward the medial side of the forearm.

Movement 2 - With the wrist, move the dumbbell laterally (away from) the midline of the body; moving the little finger side of the hand toward the lateral side of the forearm.

Movement 3- With the wrist, from a supinated position, flex the dumbbell toward your body, then go back to the starting point and repeat; this is a traditional "wrist curl."

Movement 4- With the wrist, from a pronated position, extend the dumbbell toward your body, then go back to the starting point and repeat; this is a traditional "wrist extension."

Final Thoughts

Give this routine a shot for four to six weeks and bust through your arm development stalemate!

We recommend using this routine in a bulking phase, eating a minimum of one gram of protein per pound of body weight during this phase. Abstain from alcohol and sleep a minimum of seven to eight hours nightly.

When we are training arms intensely twice a week, 72-96 hours is recommended between training sessions.

Talking time is over, lifting time begins.

The Gun Show is in town!

Time to hit the pig iron!

The Rolls Royce of Upper Chest Development

For decades, the incline press has been the go-to exercise to build the upper chest because upper chest activation is about five-percent greater when contrasted with flat benches. Activity in the front delts increases by about 80 percent.

A recent Canadian study showed that the reverse-grip bench press activated 30-percent more upper pecs than the traditional pronated/overhand grip flat bench press.

Former Muscle and Fitness Science Editor Jim Stoppani, PhD, explains: "The reverse grip helps keep your elbows in and your upper arms parallel to your torso. Moving your arms in this manner increases the use of upper pec muscle fibers."

Everything is bigger in Texas! Not surprisingly, the two most-developed upper chests ever witnessed hailed from the Lone Star State: 1990s powerlifting/bench press champions and record holders Anthony Clark and Jim Voronin. Both set records with a reverse-grip style bench press.

Here is a cluster routine to maximize "Upper Chest" Development with the reverse grip bench press

- Week 1 - do 60 % of your "regular" bench press max for four reps, rest 30 seconds, repeat this for seven minutes, last set do as many reps as possible, stopping one shy of failure.
- Week 2 - do 60 % of your "regular" bench press max for five reps, rest 30 seconds, repeat this for seven minutes, last set do as many reps as possible, stopping one shy of failure.
- Week 3 - do 60 % of your "regular" bench press max for six reps, rest 30 seconds, repeat this for seven minutes, last set do as many reps as possible, stopping one shy of failure.

Lest we Forget: Weighted Dips

In recent times, pseudo non-degreed physical therapists moonlighting as strength coaches have relentlessly tried to hijack the strength game.

Unfortunately, this cabal has tried to eradicate dips from serious muscle-building and strength training regimens.

Dips are not for the senior citizen with a shoulder replacement, BUT that doesn't mean that perfectly healthy, hardcore trainees with serious goals need to avoid what was touted by some old timers as "the upper-body squat."

As Rudyard Kipling warned ("lest we forget") about the dangers of imperial hubris in his famous poem, "Recessional," the same caveat can be issued for the arrogant belief and dismissal of proven basic exercises.

Weighted dips have helped develop some of the strongest and most muscular physiques of all time. Weighted dips have a place in a wide spectrum of programs that serve a wide range of goals.

Here are some reasons to consider adding weighted dips to your current training plan:

- MRI research, performed by Per Tesch, reported in his iconic book *Targeted Bodybuilding*, showed dips were the only movement tested that significantly stressed all three heads of the triceps.
- Bodybuilding Guru Vince Gironda claims dips are the granddaddy chest exercise. (When performed with a chin to the chest, forward lean style; upright puts greater emphasis on the triceps.)
- Weighted dips force the athlete to use his/her upper body and core to stabilize the load, unlike push-ups where the ground assists.
- Pat Casey, the first man to bench press 600 pounds, had weighted dips at the core of his program, not to mention they help the overhead press.

Athletes with shoulder or elbow injuries *may* find dips to be a good substitute for bench pressing.
Bar dips are a closed kinetic-chain exercise, unlike the bench press.

Weighted Dips Routine

Exercise	y	s	Reps	Rest	Comments
Weighted Dips	MAX	5	5	180 Sec.	Go as heavy as possible each set. After the last set, remove the added resistance as fast as possible and do as many reps possible with your bodyweight; rest 20 seconds and do as many reps as possible again with your bodyweight. Rest 20 seconds and repeat one more time.
DB Reverse Grip Bench Press	MAX	3	15	90 Sec.	Do not pace, go as heavy as possible each set, more than likely you will lower weight each subsequent set.
Clos Grip Bench Press	MAX	3	4,8,12	90 Sec.	Each weight should be to momentary muscular failure because of intensity level and increased repetitions; lower bar weight each set.
Incline Cable Flys	12-15RM	3	Failure	60 Sec.	Start with a 12-15 rep max weight; go to failure then rest 60 seconds, repeat the process twice without reducing weight.
One Armed Overhead DB Tricep Extensions	MAX	3	12	60 Sec.	Emphasize feeling the muscle work and the stretch.

Time to hit the pig iron!

Chuck Sipes — ARMageddon

Steroids emerged on the bodybuilding scene in the early 1960s; myths started to perpetuate that one no longer had to train heavy to maximize muscular development. This contradicted trial and error from the pre-steroid era, the methods of muscular supermen like Reg Park, and science.

Despite the trends, there was one holdout from the old era that believed you had to look and perform the part; this was the legendary Chuck Sipes. Chuck had some very unconventional training philosophies, but his muscularity was ahead of his time; his strength would be world-class in powerlifting even today.

Early Motivation

Growing up, Chuck dreamed of glory on the gridiron; these dreams were shattered in high school when coaches expressed Chuck was too small to make the football team.

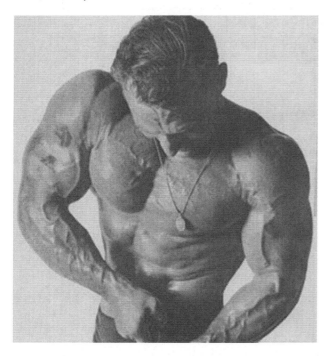

Einstein said, "Coincidence is God's way of re-maining anonymous." Coincidentally, a teenage Chuck Sipes had Chuck Coker as a neighbor. Coker is most well-known for developing *Universal Line of Equipment* and, unbeknownst to many, Peripheral Heart Action Training was Coker's brain child.

The acquisition of knowledge from Coker, repeated trial and error and unparalleled work ethic enabled Sipes to eventually bench press 570 pounds raw. The world record at the time was 617 by a man 100 pounds heavier.

In the dawn of Sipes' bodybuilding career, he worked 12-hour shifts as a lumberjack, then after work headed straight to the gym to slaughter some pig iron. Later in life, Sipes went to work with the California Youth Authority (CYA) mentoring troubled youth and giving them a new purpose with physical culture and strength training.

Overtraining or Under Working?

In a modern era, where a preponderance of neophyte trainees is paranoid about overtraining, Sipes was a total throw back using tons of sets, tons of reps, and often a ton of weight. Sipes' rest breaks between sets were generally just 10-30 seconds.

Was everything Sipes did 100-percent validated by science? Nope! But passion and consistency trump theoretical speculation in the lab every day of the week and thrice on Sunday.

Speaking of science, the mechanisms that elicit muscle hypertrophy — mechanical tension, metabolic stress and muscle damage — were exploited in the regimen of Sipes.

Chuck Sipes' Arm Specialization Routine

"The settler, the village blacksmith, the lumberjack, the carpenter…all needed powerful arms to ply their trade well, and in time those with the greatest, most powerful arms grew to be respected for their contributions,"
- Chuck Sipes

Chuck Sipes' arm development was ahead of his time.

Sipes did this workout three times weekly, but we recommend starting at one to two. Keep rest periods less than 45 seconds and continually add weight on the bar.

Chuck Sipes' ARMageddon		
Exercise	**Sets/Reps**	**Comments**
Cheat Curl	4x4	Do not heave barbell, just cheat enough to get past the sticking point, perform a three-second negative. Rest two minutes between sets.
Concentration Curl	6x8	Alternate sets in a supinated palms grip and a neutral hammer grip. Rest 90 seconds between sets.
Preacher Curl With EZ-Curl Bar	3x10	Stay very strict, rest 90 seconds between sets.
Wrist Curls/Extension	4x20	Two sets of palms up wrist curls, two sets palms down extensions for four total sets. Rest 60 seconds between sets.
Nose Crushers	4x6	Like a skull crusher but aiming point is the nose, EZ Curl or straight bar okay. Rest 90 seconds between sets.
Tricep Pushdown	3x20	Perform in a slow, methodical style, rest 60 seconds between sets.
Chin-Up Superset with Bar Dip	6x6	Perform these exercises in immediate succession; add weight to both exercises if applicable. Rest two minutes between supersets.

Go as heavy as possible on all these exercises without sacrificing form. Start heavy and decrease weight each set as needed in a reverse pyramid style.

Final Thoughts

Chuck Sipes built a base with heavy pig iron and trained with a holistic powerbuilding approach. Because of this, Sipes set a new standard of muscularity and density and was one of the first bodybuilders to have a "grainy" look.

Time to hit the pig iron!

Sipes Shoulder Explosion

Bob Hoffman (1898-1985) owned York Barbell club and was the figure of strength training and muscle building until the 1960s. Hoffman used to say, "Build the strength and the shape will follow."

By the 1960s, this adage started to disappear. Hoisting heavy weights lost its relevancy to the almighty pump. This is not all bad, as a powerbuilder trains heavy and finishes with pumping exercises, and both are essential for maximizing muscular development.

Lee Haney once said, "The key to building massive, powerful muscles is to doggedly increase the training weights you use." This even applies to pumping exercises — the keys are to never sacrifice technique, increase mechanical advantage or use momentum because you don't want to actually change the movement. You want to get stronger in all movements, but never at the expense of perfect technique.

So what changed in the 1960s?

DRUGS!

Steroids arrived on the scene in the late 1950s and in the last couple of decade's insulin, HGH and others have come along for the ride. These drugs have contributed to building physical giants in regards to muscular development, but have caused trainees to regress to mental dwarfism in regards to sound training practices.

Saying strength development does not matter in pursuit of size development is pure hogwash; science and anecdotes concur.

This workout was heavily influenced by Chuck Sipes.

Performance

Sipes loaded two barbells and performed two movements. The first exercise was very heavy; the second exercise was a pumping one. Sipes would move from exercise to exercise without delay, and we will follow his lead. We are doing the same thing, although we will include dumbbell work.

We are doing three paired exercises of four supersets each.

Sipes Shoulder Explosion - Pair 1					
Exercise	**Sets**	**Reps**	**Intensity**	**Interval**	**Comments**
Standing Overhead Press	4	2	2RM	None	*Start with a legitimate two-rep max. Lower weights on subsequent sets as needed, all sets should be as heavy as possible.*
Barbell Front Raise	4	10	10RM	None	*Start with a legitimate 10-rep max. Lower weights on subsequent sets as needed, all sets should be as heavy as possible. Do these face down on an inclined bench. Rest interval is 2-3 minutes between supersets. Take a rest for three minutes prior to starting pair 2.*

Sipes Shoulder Explosion - Pair 2

Exercise	Sets	Reps	Intensity	Rest Interval	Comments
Savickas Press	4	2	2RM	None	*Start with a legitimate two-rep max. Lower weights on subsequent sets as needed, all sets should be as heavy as possible.*
Bent Over DB Lateral Raise	4	10	10RM	None	*Start with a legitimate 10-rep max. Lower weights on subsequent sets as needed, all sets should be as heavy as possible. Do these face down on an inclined bench. Rest interval is 2-3 minutes between supersets. Take a rest for three minutes prior to starting pair 2.*

Sipes Shoulder Explosion - Pair 3

Exercise	Sets	Reps	Intensity	Rest Interval	Comments
Arnold Press	4	6	6RM	None	*Start with a legitimate six-rep max. Lower weights on subsequent sets as needed, all sets should be as heavy as possible.*
DB Incline Lateral Raise	4	10	10RM	None	*Start with a legitimate 10-rep max, use a three-second negative and emphasize the stretch at the bottom of the . Lower weights on subsequent sets as needed, all sets should be as heavy as possible. Rest interval is 2-3 minutes between supersets.*

Final Thoughts

Broad shoulders command the respect of men and melt the hearts of women. Virtually any athletic endeavor will benefit from stronger shoulders.

Time to hit the pig iron!

Old School Norseman Training

In the late 1990s, where I grew up in Southern California, hardcore, old-school training regimens of Arnold, Franco, and Bill Pearl had given way to flushing routines on the smith machine, spandex and synthol.

The old-time bodybuilders like Pearl and Grimek supplemented their incomes by performing extraordinary feats of strength, while others worked as debt collectors or doormen at illegal drinking pens. These cats were all around bad-asses

I heard stories about the old timers from some of the Old Heads at the YMCA. It was a relief, because I knew there was more to physical culture than spandex, chrome machines and artificially-pumped muscles.

A Crisis Produces Opportunity.

My struggle led me to endless research on the history of the iron game. One individual that I learned of that inspired me was Karl "The Noble Norseman" Norberg. In college, I wrote a paper on Norberg; unfortunately, my professor did not see the nobility of this pumped-up Swedish Stevedore.

I have a feeling you will.

The Noble Norsemen

Karl Norberg was the strongest longshoreman of all time. He was born in Sweden on January 5, 1893. By 12 years old, Norberg, one of a dozen siblings, worked at a sawmill 12 hours a day, generally six days a week.

Norberg continued working manual labor jobs and eventually migrated to the United States in 1927. With no pretense of trading in his blue collar for a white one, Norberg found his calling as a longshoreman in San Francisco. Long before the days of forklifts, overtime, mandatory breaks and other labor rights, Norberg worked around the clock every day of the week.

From day one on the docks, The Noble Norseman dazzled coworkers and passersby with amazing feats of strength he acquired from years of "strongman training" a.k.a. heavy manual labor.

Grimek Meets Norberg

John Grimek, a forefather of modern bodybuilding, had an extensive strength background like other greats prior to chemical warfare. This background went beyond strength feats at travelling carnivals. Grimek was a national weightlifting champion and even competed in the Olympics. In those days, the overhead press was contested as an Olympic lift, and this was Grimek's forte.

Fast forward to 1941, the esteemed John Grimek was performing an overhead press exhibition in San Franciso. Norberg and a few of the booze hounds from the ship yard went down to check it out. The dockworkers began to heckle Grimek and faithfully believed one of their own could defeat him. After all, Norberg was functionally strong and had begun a weight-training regimen.

Putting things in perspective, a 31-year-old Grimek was in his prime; Norberg was two years away from getting his AARP card and, furthermore, lacked any formal instruction.

Norberg was reluctant to go against Grimek at first, but once he saw John was up for it, it was on like Donkey Kong!

The most Norberg had ever pressed was 255, and the contest ensued at opening weight of 240 pounds. Initially, Norberg matched Grimek attempt-by-attempt. Eventually, Grimek ended up winning with a 280-pound press, while Norberg made a 270-pound press. Norberg nearly defeated Grimek — even more impressive, Norberg cheat-curled the barbell to chest level, then switched from an underhand to an overhand grip at chest level and pressed the weight overhead.

Grimek had nearly met his match. This would be akin to an unknown 50-year-old street fighter losing to a top UFC Champion by split decision in the octagon.

Norberg Defies Age Limits

Like a fine Bourbon, as Norberg aged, he improved! At 74 years young, he performed a double with 460 pounds in the bench press and held a pair of 80-pound dumbbells straight out from his body in a crucifix style. At 80, Norberg benched 400 pounds.

One of two other impressive and less-documented lifts, according to Jeff Everson of *Planet Muscle,* was a deadlift of 600 pounds made after the age of 65. This was the first time he tried the lift! Years of heavy loading had paid off, Norberg walked with the barbell after locking the weight out. In addition, he hit a seated Military Press with 325 pounds.

Noble Norseman Training Routine

Karl did this routine three days a week. He did not train legs heavy because of severe arthritis in his knees and hips:

The Noble Norsmen Routine		
Exercise	**Sets**	**Reps**
Bench	3	*Work up to 6RM, then 3RM, Then 1RM*
Behind the Neck Press	3	*Work up to 6RM, then 3RM, Then 1RM*
Incline	3	*Work up to 6RM, then 3RM, Then 1RM*
Dumbbell Rows	5	*Multiple Rep Ranges*

Final Thoughts

Michelangelo said, *"The greater danger for most of us lies not in setting our aim too high and falling short; but in setting our aim too low, and achieving our mark."*

Not Norberg!

The mighty longshoreman grabbed the bull by the testicles and spit in the face of preconceived age-notions.

Norberg is a legend, an inspiration and cannot be forgotten; it is important to pay tribute to our forefathers in the iron game.

Time to hit the pig iron!

Pre-Exhaust Shoulder Training

Compound movements equal compound results! Big movements produce big results! Okay, okay, we get it!

Because compound movements are neurologically and physically more demanding than isolation movements, a good rule of thumb is to perform heavy compound movements first in a training session via a powerbuilding or post-exhaust approach.

This rule has to hold true a majority of the time if acquisition of strength and muscle mass is the training objective. However, it's a mere guideline and there is a time and a place to break it.

Doing the same thing over and over and expecting a different result is the definition of insanity.

With this routine, we are going to take a break from the heavy powerbuilding and hammer out a pre-exhaust routine.

This is not a vacation — it's introducing a painful, fun and effective new stimulus.

Pre-Exhaust Defined

What is pre-exhaust training? Using a single-joint "isolation" movement to failure before performing a heavier multi-joint "compound" movement is called pre-exhaustion training. A practical example would be leg extensions before front squats (for the quadriceps) or cable flys before the bench press for the chest.

This technique was popularized by Arnold Schwarzenegger in the movie *Pumping Iron*. If you watched it, you'll remember Arnold performing leg extensions before squats. The theory behind pre-exhaustion training is that when you fatigue the prime mover-muscle with an isolation exercise prior to a heavier compound movement, the supporting muscles are no longer the limiting factor. Oftentimes, when squatting, the lower back is the limiting factor and not the legs! The idea with pre-exhaust training is to fatigue the legs before squats, so squats adequately stimulate the legs in their weakened and fatigued state.

Some prominent coaches and trainers believe pre-exhaustion training is friendlier on the joints. The idea is, as muscular fatigue sets in, prior to training heavy compound movements, these movements can now be trained using lighter loads yet still yield hypertrophic benefits.

Why Pre-Exhaust?

The Repeated Bout Effect (RBE), in a nutshell, says doing the same exercises over and over will cause less muscle damage (a key variable in the muscle growth equation) over time. Essentially, one adapts. One way to throw a monkey wrench at RBE is with pre-exhaust training.

Since we are focusing on shoulders this workout, this can serve as a remedial course in reestablishing the mind-muscle connection with shoulders. The anecdotes of top bodybuilders suggest that concentrating and purposeful recruitment of the particular muscle one is intending to work more effectively targets that muscle (ex: feeling your side delts work when performing a lateral raise).

Research confirms this!

This pre-exhaust routine is going to give you a chance to rekindle the mind-muscle connection. This will not happen on heavy sets of five in the military press, nor should it. We are starting off with isolation exercises to rekindle that old flame.

Joint pain! Many lifters' elbows could use a break from heavy pressing by starting the workout with lighter isolation movements; pressing movements will not need to be performed as heavy to stimulate the shoulders.

Finally, it's fun to change things up; a new workout provides a new challenge. We are going to pay homage to former *MuscleMag* Publisher, the late Robert Kennedy, who popularized pre-exhaust training in 1968 when he first publicized it to the masses.

The Pre Exhaust Routine			
Exercise	**Sets**	**Reps**	**Comments**
Incline DB Lateral Raise- Standing DB Lateral Raise	3	12/??	*Start with a weight you can do 12 reps with on on incline dumbbell lateral raise, do it to failure and keep perfect technique. Emphasize the stretch at the bottom of the movement; otherwise it's a wasted movement. After failure is reached, immediately do the same weights to failure on the standing dumbbell lateral raise. Hold the contracted position for one second. Reduce weight 20 percent each superset, rest two minutes between supersets.*
Reverse DB Fly	3	15	*Emphasize technique. Do each set with as much weight possible, keeping in mind range of motion is more important than the weight being used. Torso should be parallel to the floor, hold the top contracted position for half a second, rest 75 seconds between sets.*
DB Front Raise	3	12/??	*The dumbbell front raises; should be strict holding the top contracted position at top half of a second. Start with a weight you can do 12 reps with on the front raises, do it to failure and keep perfect technique. After failure is reached, immediately perform hand stand push-ups to failure. Reduce weight 20 percent each superset on front raises, use bodyweight each set of hand stand push-ups, rest two minutes between supersets. (If you are unable to do a handstand push-up try the downward dog variation)*
Face Pulls	3	15	*Pick the maximum weight you can use for 15 repetitions, maintain perfect form. Cheating this exercise cheats you out of the intended benefits. Emphasize a full range of motion and hold the contracted position for one second. This exercise as demonstrated through EMG (measuring the electrical activity of muscle) not only hits the posterior aspect of the shoulders as expected but significantly hits the side portion. Take a one-minute rest between sets.*
Standing Overhead Press	3	6	*In the overhead press, you will be fatigued, but still go as heavy as possible, rest two minutes between sets.*

Pre-Exhaust Chest Routine

Since we are focusing on chest this workout, think about lifters with disproportionately strong triceps and shoulders, it may be tough to receive adequate chest stimulation with traditional pressing movements.

Pre-exhaust training can help these lifters receive adequate chest stimulation; furthermore, many folks could use a break from heavy chest-pressing variations.

Pre-Exhaust Chest Routine			
Exercise	**Sets**	**Reps**	**Comments**
Cable Incline Fly/Cable Decline Fly	3	12/??	Start with a weight you can do 12 reps with on an incline fly, do it to failure and keep perfect technique. After failure is reached immediately do the same weight to failure on a decline fly. Hold the contracted position for one second. Reduce weight 20 percent each superset. Rest two minutes between supersets.
Flat DB Fly	3	15	Emphasize stretch and technique. Do each set with as much weight possible, keeping in mind range of motion is more important than the weight being used. Rest 75 seconds between sets
Standing Uppercut Fly/Push Up	3	12/??	Perform upper cut flys standing between cables; hold contracted position at top for one second. Start with a weight you can do 12 reps with on an uppercut fly, do it to failure and keep perfect technique. After failure is reached, immediately perform push-ups to failure. Reduce weight 20 percent each superset on flys, use bodyweight each set of push-ups. Rest two minutes between supersets.
Reverse Grip Bench DB	1	MAX	Pick a weight that is 15 percent of your bench press max in each hand. If you can bench press 300 pounds, use 45 pound dumbbells. At a steady tempo, perform as many reps as possible for 90 seconds at failure continue with partials. Do not drop the dumbbells no matter what, even if they are moving a quarter inch.
Bench Press	3	6	In the bench press, you will be fatigued, but still go as heavy as possible. Rest two minutes between sets.

A Call to Arms

Big arms command respect from the Scotland Yard to the prison yard — not to mention garner prolonged feminine stares at your kid's little league game or the local community pool.

Far too many folks drink the Kool Aid of all that matters is "the pump" when training arms, pumping out set after set using very high reps with pygmy weights. Sure, the pump matters, but when it comes to arm development, there is no way to circumvent heavy-ass pig iron.

We are going to have you in and out of the gym in 40 minutes with a purposeful path to an arm-growth Valhalla.

Dips

From the biggest "back arms" on the prison tier to old-school bodybuilding legends like Reg Park and modern day behemoths like the greatest bodybuilder of all-time, Ronnie Coleman, dips were a mainstay.

The strongest overhead pressers and bench pressers to walk the face of the earth have trained dips.

We are not talking about some short range of motion, cutesy bench dips—we are talking about old-school, blood and guts parallel-bar dips.

Besides the anecdotes, dips were the only exercise that provided significant overload to all three heads of the triceps as demonstrated by MRI scans in Per Tesch's epic classic *Targeted Bodybuilding.*

Because triceps make up 2/3 of the upper arm, we will start with what's most important first and commence with dips.

We will do three sets of five reps, adding weight if possible. For the first two sets, do a weight you are capable of doing six to eight reps with; on the final set go to failure. Upon failure, do two more dips, step back up to the extended position and lower yourself for a steady five-second tempo until reaching the bottom position (arms parallel to the floor).

We can do more eccentrically so we will — the goal is to build as much muscle as fast as possible.

Important Notes: Stay as upright as possible to keep emphasis on triceps.

Hercules Chin-Up

The Hercules chin-up is a creation of the Jailhouse Strong training system that uses incremental movements to build Herculean biceps. Pull yourself up until your chin is over the bar and hold for two seconds. Then, descend halfway down and hold for two seconds. Then repeat this movement for the prescribed number of repetitions. Finish with arms fully extended at the bottom.

Do this for three sets of four reps, adding weight if possible.

Do this immediately after dips and rest two minutes after each superset.

Important Notes: Make sure your chin is completely over the bar and focus intentionally on the bicep contraction.

Dicks Press

This tricep movement was developed by legendary powerlifter Paul Dicks. It is a favorite for slapping slabs of meat on the triceps among bodybuilders.

Do this movement for three sets of six- to eight-reps as heavy as possible while maintaining great technique.

Important Notes: Lower the weight to approximately one inch above your chest, push your elbows up and shift the bar toward your chin. Then shift the bar back to one inch above your chest, forcefully press up and repeat.

Incline Dumbbell Curls

For generations, strength athletes have increased strength with extended range-of-motion movements like deficit deadlifts, cambered bar bench presses and Olympic pause squats to build strength. Smart bodybuilders have maximized muscularity by including extended range-of-motion movements. These movements prolong time under tension and cause greater muscle damage (a good thing for hypertrophy).

For the biceps, look no further than the incline bicep curl for extending your range of motion. Do this for three sets of six reps as heavy as possible.

Important notes: Hold each rep in the bottom position for one second, emphasizing the stretch. Hold weight for one second in top contracted position. Range of motion should never be sacrificed for weight.

Finisher

Since triceps are the key to arm growth, we will finish just like we started by giving the triceps a brutal beat down.

We will do bodyweight triceps extensions. With bodyweight exercises, decrease mechanical advantage to increase difficulty. In this case, the further your feet are from the bar you are grasping with your hands, the more difficult the movement — the more elevated the feet, the more difficult the movement.

The path of least resistance is the path of the least results, so be honest with yourself.

We will use the total repetition method, meaning we will achieve the desired number of reps in the fewest number sets possible. Using the total repetition method, 100 triceps extensions might look something like this: *Set 1 - 15 reps, Set 2 - 12 reps, Set 3 - 11 reps, Set 4 -10 reps, Set 5 - 10 reps, Set 6 - 9 reps, Set 7 - 8 reps, Set 8 - 7 reps, Set 9 - 7 reps, Set 10 - 6 reps, Set 11 - 5 reps.*

Your goal is to complete 100 repetitions inside of 10 minutes. Rest as needed. At 10 minutes you stop regardless of whether you completed the 100 reps or not — time is of the essence.

Final Thoughts

Big arms fascinate the lay public and the hardcore bodybuilding aficionado alike. If your arms have not grown since Reagan was in office you have to try something different —give this fast, effective routine a shot; you have nothing to lose!

Time to hit the pig iron!

No Time, No Problem — The Ultimate Chest Slay

People generally do what's most important first. The first day of the week, Monday, is known as international chest day in the commercial gym world. We can debate the merits of what's most important til' the cows come home — regardless of the debate, no other body part has received its own "unofficial day."

Behind bars, the chest is referred to as "the hood." A well-developed "hood" is a status symbol on the prison yard weight pile.

Bodybuilders that lack suitable chest development are often accused of "disappearing" when turning to the side… not a good thing.

Bottom line: anyone from the hedge fund manager to the bouncer at the local kick-n-stab, can garner respect from a well-developed chest.

We know your time is limited — you may not have access to all of the latest "advancements" in chrome machines. If you are willing to work hard once a week, we can help take your chest development to a whole new level.

The Reverse-Grip Bench Press

Lots of bodybuilding methods are based off tradition; let's buck tradition and turn to science to take your upper-chest development to a whole new level. If the lab ain't your thing, here is a powerful anecdote: the two biggest upper chests ever witnessed were by Texas Powerlifting Titans Big Jim Voronin and the late Anthony Clark. Both trained and competed with the reverse-grip bench press.

Unconventional training strategies can yield unconventional results — a good thing if you want to break away from the pack. Most people have problems with the upper chest, so that's where we'll start.

A recent Canadian study showed that the reverse-grip bench press increased upper pec activation by 30 percent compared to a traditional/flat pronated-grip bench press. Comparatively, incline has about five-percent greater upper-pec activation over the traditional bench presses.

For the reverse-grip bench press, when warming up, we are going to perform the exercise for 10 minutes using cluster sets with 65 percent of your regular-grip bench press max for four reps. Rest 30 seconds and repeat this process until 10 minutes is reached; on the last set, if you have any gas left, complete as many repetitions as possible.

Tips: Make sure you use a spotter to lift the bar off, thumbs around the bar (much more risky than a traditional bench press) and if you cannot get the technique right, try dumbbells.

Dumbbell Pullover

The dumbbell pullover was a favorite of some of the greatest chests of all time, like Arnold Schwarzenegger and Reg Park. This exercise works not only the chest but also the lats and the intercostal serratus anterior (the muscles of the ribcage).

Maximally developed intercostal muscles will give the illusion of a bigger rib cage when taking a deep breath and holding a pose because the ribs are pulled up by the intercostal muscles

After each exercise, complete one set of 15 reps of dumbbell pullovers with a moderately light weight, emphasizing the stretch.

Important notes: Do this with a movement intention style, focusing on the stretch, and feeling the movement while keeping reps in the 12+ range.

If you have a history of shoulder problems, be careful when introducing this exercise. You may need to avoid it altogether.

Dips

Bodybuilding guru, the late Vince Gironda, felt dips were the best movement for stimulating muscle growth in the upper body. Virtually every great bodybuilder, from the classical era to the modern-day pros, has included dips in the training regimen. The same holds true for the strongest raw bench-pressers of all time.

Dips will be performed for five sets of five repetitions, progressively adding weight each set if possible. After the last set, remove the added resistance as fast as possible and do as many reps as possible with your bodyweight; rest 20 seconds and do as many reps as possible again with your bodyweight. Rest 20 seconds and repeat one more time. The rest interval is 90 seconds between working set of dips.

Tips: Lean forward to place emphasis on your chest.

Cable Flys

We are going to opt for cables at this point because your stabilizing muscles are tired and cables provide continuous resistance throughout the entire range of motion. Focus needs to be on a full range of motion. Perform the negative portion of each rep for three seconds; perform the positive forcefully, holding the peak-contracted position at the top for a second.

Pick a weight with which you can do 12-15 reps. Perform the reps in the fashion described for one minute straight. If you fail before a minute, continue the set with partials and do not stop — start with perfect form and end by any means necessary! Rest two minutes and then do the same thing for 40 seconds. Rest two minutes and the final set will be completed for 30 seconds.

Finisher

We are going to finish with five minutes of push-ups. Perform push-ups to failure, rest 30 seconds, then repeat the process until you hit five minutes. Failure means failure, not discomfort! Get the most out of it.

Final Thoughts

The old cliché "you are only cheating yourself" applies to anyone that doesn't give 100 percent on this workout — half-assed effort will simply equate to half-assed results. On the other hand, developing the functional power to push your way through the BS at the next sales convention or build a powerful looking "hood" can be accomplished with this workout.

Time to hit the pig iron!

Ultimate Chest Slay

Exercise	Sets/Reps	Intensity	Rest Interval
Reverse Grip Bench Press	Max X 4	*65%*	30 Sec.
DB Pullovers	1x15 (After Each Exercise)	*Light*	
Dips	5x5 RP	*MAX*	90 Sec.
Cable Flys	3x MAX	*12-15RM*	120 Sec.
Push Up	5 Min.		

■ ■ ■

Lumberjack Forearms

For centuries, the quality of a blacksmith was judged by the quality of his forearm development.

Extreme forearm development is intimidating and impressive. A legitimately strong individual proudly wears well-developed forearms, like a knight wears armor. A solid grip is a badge of honor and well-developed forearms shout functional power.

The lucky ones have impressive forearms without doing any direct forearm work, while the rest of us will need direct training to maximally develop the forearms.

Powerbuilding legend Anthony Ditillo had this to say about his massive increase in forearm size and how he trained his forearms in 1969:

> *"I train my forearms 4 times per week; twice at the end of my upper-body training days and again twice at the onset of my lower-body training days. I perform the Reverse Curl first, doing 5 sets of 10-8-6-4-15 repetitions using progressively heavier weights each set (excepting the last). I then perform the seated wrist curl, palms up, for 5 additional sets of 20 repetitions using the same weight, increasing it whenever possible. I also followed proper diet principles."*

In the tradition of Ditillo, we will train our forearms four days a week using low and high reps and a variety of exercises. These workouts can be done as an addendum to current training sessions or in separate workouts.

Forearm Blast				
Day	**Exercise**	**Sets**	**Reps**	**Comments**
Day 1	**Towel Hangs**	2	30 Sec.	*Drape a towel over the top of a squat rack, hold the bottom of the towel for 30 seconds; if this is easy, add weight--this should be very difficult. Unable to use a towel? Hang on a pull-up bar. Rest two minutes between sets.*
	Cheat Reverse Curls	5	5 (5 Sec. Negative)	*Go as heavy as possible; use Fat Gripz, if available. It is okay to use momentum on the way up; the work is on the way down. Rest 90 seconds between sets.*
Day 2	**Wrist Curl**	4	15	*Exercises to be done in a superset fashion. Rest 1-2 Min between supersets.*
	Wrist Extension	4	15	
Day 3	**DB Ulnar Deviation**	4	15	*With wrist, move dumbbell toward the midline of the body; moving the little finger side of the hand toward the medial side of the forearm. Go as heavy as possible; use strict form this is an isolation exercise. Rest 60 seconds between sets.*
	Radial Deviation	4	15	*With wrist, move dumbbell laterally (away from) the midline of the body; moving the little finger side of the hand toward the lateral side of the forearm. Go as heavy as possible; use strict form this is an isolation exercise. Rest 60 seconds between sets*
Day 4	**Captains of Crush Gripper**	8	See Description	*For six minutes straight we are going to build function crush grip, while adding slabs of muscle to the forearms. Using a captain crush gripper or any squeeze grip machine—start off with resistance that could be performed for 15 reps. Perform six reps on your weaker side, getting a full range of motion; repeat on the stronger side for six reps. When you can no longer do six reps on the weaker side go to five, when five is no longer possible go to four, when four is no longer possible go to three, when three is no longer possible go to two and when two is no longer possible go to one. If one is no longer possible, squeeze the gripper as hard as possible for five seconds, continually matching the strong side reps to those first accomplished on the weak side. No rest between sets.*
	Reverse Drag Curl	4	10,8,6,5	*With a shoulder width pronated grip on a loaded barbell, let the weight hang in your hands and slowly drag the barbell up your body as high as you can get it and then back down again. Want to increase difficulty? Use Fat Gripz or wrap a towel around the barbell*

Final Thoughts

Huge forearms are part of the reason no one anytime soon will defeat Flex Lewis for the under 212-pound Olympia crown.

Huge forearms make lifters look the part and functionally contribute to extraordinary feats of strength.

Time to hit the pig iron!

Delt Drudgery

Broad shoulders project an image of strength and masculinity that gives the waist a smaller, tapered look. There is just something special about big, wide shoulders that intrigues women and intimidates men.

Beyond the aesthetic appeal, strong, developed shoulders play a role in pretty much any upper body movement that requires strength and power.

To maximally develop the shoulders requires a holistic approach that uses fast and slow tempos, a variety of rep ranges, compound and isolation movements.

If you promise to give us all-out effort, we will give you a great workout that will get you in and out of the gym in less than 45 minutes.

Overhead Presses

Until 1972, the standing overhead press was contested in the Olympics. Before the bench press, the standing press is what strength aficionados and the lay public accepted as the standard of upper-body strength.

Overhead presses serve to build masculine brawn, enhance utilitarian strength, and fulfill the traditional look of raw power.

For overhead presses, complete three sets of five reps. On the first two sets, use a weight you are capable of doing six to eight reps with; on the third set go to failure. At failure, push-press the weight for three additional reps and lower the weight back to the starting point with a five-second eccentric. This is an eccentric-emphasis mechanical drop-set in action.

Rest Interval: 180 Seconds

Important Notes: Do not do a standing incline press. Make sure to push your head through when locking out the weight in order to work the entire shoulder.

Incline Dumbbell Lateral Raises

Lateral raises focus on the medial/side delts, the part of the shoulder that gives the appearance of width. Lie back on an incline bench and hold the dumbbells at your sides like suitcases. Keep a 10-15 degree bend in your elbow throughout the entirety of the movement, and perform by lifting your arms out to your sides until the dumbbells are at shoulder level.

Lower the dumbbells back to the starting position using a four-second negative. Repeat this movement for eight reps. Perform three sets going as heavy as possible without sacrificing tempo or range of motion.

Lots of bodybuilders do heavy lateral raises relying on momentum. For this movement, concentrate on feeling the side delts doing the work. This is called muscle intention.

Because of the incline, this is an extended range-of-motion movement, so time under tension is prolonged and a larger amount of muscle damage results (a good thing for hypertrophy).

Rest Interval: 60 seconds

Important note: Cue the muscle working, not the movement; this is not an ego lift.

Face Pull — Bent over Lateral Raise Superset

Face pulls work the posterior deltoid and, surprisingly to most, even put extreme stress on the medial deltoid according to EMG studies. Furthermore, face pulls target your back's weak scapular muscles, which aid in stabilization of your shoulder joints. This is great for shoulder health. Additionally, this movement strengthens your lower traps.

Do this for three sets of 12 reps.

Important note: Keep this exercise strict. Hold contracted position for one second. Bands or a pulley will work.

With no rest, immediately hit bent-over lateral raises. This will be done for three sets of 15 reps. This movement directly targets the posterior delt, or the back of the shoulders.

Rest Interval: 90 seconds between Supersets

Important note: Keep this movement strict. One variation you can do is to make the movement head supported, putting your forehead on the back of an incline bench to make sure your torso position doesn't change.

Around the Worlds

A fatiguing finisher — hurts so good!

Hold a plate with your hands just in front of your abs, elbows just shy of extension. With the elbow in this fixed position, lift the weight around your head in a clock wise motion for 12 reps. Repeat the motion for 12 reps counter clockwise, and finally finish with 12 front plate raises to forehead level. This is one set.

On the second set do this for nine reps in all three directions, and for the final sets do six reps in all three directions. Your delts will feel like they can bust seams in button up shirts!

Rest Interval: 60 seconds

Important note: Keep this movement strict as long as possible. Once failure has been reached using strict technique, a moderate cheat is permitted to get the weight up. However, from the top down make sure to control the eccentric.

Delt Drudgery				
Exercise	**Sets**	**Reps**	**Intensity**	**Rest Interval**
Overhead Press	3	5,5,MAX	See Description	180 Sec.
Incline DB Lateral Raise	3	8	See Description	60 Sec.
Face Pull/Bent Over Lateral Raise Superset	3	12--15	See Description	90 Sec.
Around the Worlds	3	12,9,6	See Description	60 Sec.

Final Thoughts

"I ask not for a lighter burden, but for broader shoulders,"
- Old Jewish proverb

The functionality of building ridiculously strong shoulders is a crucial component of a workout program for cage fighters, strongmen, doormen, rugged outdoorsmen, Hawaiian watermen, and even pumped-up cons on the jailhouse yard.

For the aesthetic-minded individual, this means a tapered-looking waist and a persona of power. Bottom line: big, strong shoulders suit almost any physical goal and project confidence.

Time to hit the pig iron!

Dublin Doorman Chest

Powerbuilding is a hybrid of bodybuilding and powerlifting training and has nothing to do with competing.

In bodybuilding's genesis, athletes were required to perform strength feats with posing routines. Strength is your base for everything, including aesthetics; building pure power will require some bodybuilding movements.

Big movements produce big results; core movements must form the core of your training program even if pure aesthetics is the goal.

Examples are squat variations, bench press variations, deadlift variations, dips and pull-up variations; these movements build the most muscle mass and produce the highest levels of inter- and intra-muscle coordination and High Threshold Motor Unit (HTMU) recruitment, which has the highest potential for growth. These movements also cause your body to release greater amounts of anabolic hormones than machines or single-joint movements.

Rep ranges have to vary. Sets with lower reps (fewer than six) cause myofibrillar hypertrophy; this is the contractile element of the muscle that makes you stronger, but from an aesthetic standpoint makes a muscle look dense. Bodybuilders that never lift heavy with low reps do not have that dense, grainy look when dieted down.

Sarcoplasmic hypertrophy is the result of higher reps; this is almost like swelling up the muscle. It's the non-contractile element; this does not make you stronger. For the athlete confined to a weight class, this is like increasing the size of a car with no increase in engine size — not a good thing! For the bodybuilder, it is essential to fully develop a muscle.

All rep ranges need to be trained! Isolation exercises will also play a role. Core movements are more functional and natural but to supernaturally develop certain muscles, you will need to overload them with principle of isolation. Let's look at the vastus lateralis, or the sweep of the quads. To fully develop it, you have to do leg extensions. No human movements isolate the quads from the hamstrings, but a large sweep is the standard, so to acquire the sweep, you have to step outside the functional training paradigm and hit the leg extensions.

A holistic training approach is needed to maximally develop your physique!

This is powerbuilding!

Powerbuilding Chest Routine

Exercise	Sets	Reps	Comments
Bench Press	2	RP	Load 85 percent of your one-repetition max on the barbell. Lift the weight for as many reps as possible, take a 20-second rest interval, and do the same weight again; this will probably be two to three repetitions. Repeat this process twice, for a total of three mini sets. On the second set, use 75 percent of your one-repetition max. Take a three-minute rest interval between sets
DIP	3	6,6,MAX w/ Eccentric Emphasis	Lean forward on dips to shift the emphasis to your chest. Perform two sets of six reps with your eight-repetition max weight. On the final set go to failure, then complete two more reps with just the negative, draw each negative out for five seconds. . Take a two-minute rest interval between sets.
Reverse Grip DB Bench Press	3	6,8,12	EMG studies show this exercises emphasizes the musculature of the upper pecs much more effectively than incline presses. Perform each set as heavy as possible. Take a 90-second rest interval between sets.
Incline Cable Flys	3	12	Emphasize the stretch and hold the contraction for one second at the top of the movement, think muscle not movement. Take a one-minute rest interval between sets.
DB Bench Press	1	90 Sec.	Perform a slow, rhythmic style one to two seconds on the positive and two to three seconds on the negative. Do not drop the dumbbells, if thy stop moving, hold a static contraction or continue with partials.
Push Ups		Juarez Valley 12	The Juarez Valley Method is a creation of the Jailhouse Strong System and offers alternating ascending and descending reps. Repetitions are performed in descending order on all odd-number sets, but repetitions are performed in ascending order on even-number sets. In the middle, they meet! A Juarez Valley 12 is performed liked this: Set 1-12 reps, Set 2-1 rep, Set3-11 reps, Set 4-2 reps, Set 5-10 reps, Set 6-3 reps, Set 7-9 reps, Set 8-4 reps, Set 9-8 reps, Set 10-5 reps, Set 11-7 reps, Set 12-6 Reps

Size & Strength--Chest Routine

Bodybuilding arm and leg development from the 1960s and 70s pales in comparison to the modern era. Over the same span of decades, in spite of the introduction of space-age drugs that make Dianabol look benign, chest development has digressed.

The hubris of modern day gurus to promote gimmicks and abandon the use of bench press for chest development is frightening — how is it possible that modern day bodybuilders weighing 50 pounds more than their classical counterparts, carrying less body fat, have weaker chest development?

It's the abandonment of power!

We are going to buck the establishment and build the chest with this powerbuilding routine that has the bench press at its nucleus. If it's good enough for Arnold Schwarzenegger, it's good enough for us.

Anyone with a shred of muscular development from weight training commonly gets asked, "How much ya bench?"

A big bench press serves as your manhood in high school, part of the NFL combine test and, in the 1970s, even as an initiation tool into prison gangs.

"Functional" training advocates love to rag on the bench press for transference to sport and even hypertrophy. Generally, people with this attitude suck at the lift and carry about as much muscle as the average tin can.

These arm chair academics need to heed the words of the existentialist philosopher Jean-Paul Sarte, *"Only the guy who isn't rowing has time to rock the boat."* In other words, put down the damn test tubes and start lifting some barbells.

The greatest bodybuilder of all-time, Ronnie Coleman, had the bench press at the nucleus of his chest-training routine; Ronnie can toy with five plates for multiple reps on the bench press.

Arnold Schwarzenegger, who arguably had the greatest chest development of all-time, like Ronnie, started as a powerlifter. Furthermore, before personal training was a recognized profession, "The Austrian Oak" hired Lone Star Powerlifting legend Doug Young as a mass building consultant; Young held the bench press world record for decades.

We discussed already why the bench press has gotten a bad rap from the functional crowd—the other reason for the bad rap is the bench press shirt. Some powerlifters compete in contests that allow bench press shirts that can add up to 500 pounds to "their" lift. To each their own, but this completely robs the musculature of work and the physique of development.

We are going to train to get stronger, but, of course, put those final bodybuilding touches the powerlifts lack with this powerbuilding routine.

Powerbuilding Chest Routine 2			
Exercise	**Sets**	**Reps**	**Comments**
Bench Press	4	2,4,6,12	*Control the negative and perform the positive as explosively as possible. Each set should be as heavy as possible without sacrificing form. Take a three-minute rest interval between sets.*
Reverse Grip Bench Press	4	5,6,6,15	*EMG studies show that the reverse grip bench press activates the upper pec region better than incline presses while reducing shoulder involvement. Control the negative and perform the positive as explosively as possible. Each set should be as heavy as possible without sacrificing form. Take a two-minute rest interval between sets.*
Decline DB Press	2	TUT	*Perform a three-second negative and then perform the positive as explosively as possible. Pick a weight you can do 12-14 reps with--then do as many reps as possible for 60 seconds once you reach failure continue with partials. DO NOT DROP THE DUMBBELLS, even if the weight is moving a millimeter, for the second set reduce the weight by 1/3. Take a two-minute rest interval between sets*
Cable Flys/Push Up Superset	3	12/Failure	*This a superset, perform the cable flyes on a flat bench, using a three-second negative and holding the contracted position for one second, bend your elbows 10 degrees and keep this angle constantly through the entire movement. Focus on the stretch at the bottom of the movement and feeling the pecs working. After 12 reps of cable flyes, immediately perform push-ups to failure. Rest two minutes between superset*

Final Thoughts

Maximizing muscle hypertrophy requires going heavy, doing a variety rep ranges and tempos. Our objective with powerbuilding is to make you strong but also look the part. We are leaving no stone unturned.

Time to hit the pig iron!

Rest-Pause Drops

Behind bars, in the Rockview Penitentiary, Jim Williams used a variation of the rest-pause method to build a bench press over 40 years ago that only a few people on the planet could duplicate even today.

IFBB Pro Michael Christian would train on three bench presses. He would start with a weight he could bench press for 8-10 reps, take a slight break and try to match the reps on the next bench, take a slight rest and do the same thing on the next bench.

This is the rest-pause method in action!

Despite not taking the Weider "company line," Christian was a Mr. Olympia runner-up.

While it's clear in correctional institutions that rest-pause training is beloved, institutes of higher learning confirm its efficiency.

One study published in *Journal of Science & Medicine In Sport* in 2012 showed a rest-pause group, when compared to a traditional-set workout and a cluster-set workout, recruited more motor units, completed the same work in less time and didn't cause any greater post-workout fatigue.

One study published in *Journal of Translational Medicine* found that a rest-pause training protocol with less volume and the same load was accomplished in nearly half the time of a traditional resistance training program. However, the post-workout resting energy expenditure was much greater with the rest-pause group. In a nutshell, the group that trained rest-pause style was burning more calories at rest than those training in a traditional style for a full day after their final rep.

In summary, rest-pause training allows one to get more done in less time.

Applied

Rest-pause training breaks down one set into several sub-sets with a brief rest between each. For this workout you will load a weight you can perform for 6-10 repetitions, lift the weight for as many reps as possible, take a 20-second rest interval, and do the same weight again; this will probably be two to three repetitions. Repeat this process twice; for a total of three sub-sets.

Looking at the bench press, a rest-pause series might look something like this:

Set 1: 250x8 reps
Rest 20 seconds
Set 2: 250x3 reps
Rest 20 seconds
Set 3: 250x2 reps

Drop Sets

Drops sets have been an integral part of the muscle-building regimens of bodybuilders ranging from Larry Scott to Branch Warren.

Drop sets work simply because they recruit the entire spectrum of muscle fibers, ranging from the powerful fast-twitch fibers down to the slow-twitch fibers.

Drop sets have been used as a way to continue exercise with lighter weights and maximal intensity once muscular failure has been reached. This in turn stimulates the release of growth hormone (GH) and insulin-like growth factor-1 (IGF-1).

Practically Applied

Using the dumbbell incline press as an example with a pair of 100s, you would perform this weight until failure. Next, you would do the same thing with 80s then finish with 60s.

Barbell drop-sets are usually associated with the strip set, meaning you have small plates on the barbell and, once muscular failure is reached, you strip one of the plates off and continue.

An example would be doing triceps extensions with 105 pounds, which would be a 45-pound bar with three 10s on each side; curl this weight until failure. Then, your partners immediately strip a 10-pound plate off each side and you do 85 pounds until muscle failure. Repeat the process, and then it is 65 pounds until failure. You could continue this all the way down to the 45-pound Olympic bar.

Generally, drop sets are reduced in weight/intensity 10- to 30-percent per drop, and two to three drops are performed.

Rest-Pause Drop Combo

Bodybuilding gurus say you can train long (high volume), or intense. Combining these two methods, we can get an intense workout without skimping on the volume.

Once you are warmed up, we are going to have you in and out in 30 minutes; this requires a 100-percent physical effort and 100-percent mental focus — no Facebook updates, no social interaction period. As our friend Ray Toulany says, *"To truly see a man train hard is frightening."*

What Is a Rest-Pause Drop (RPD)?

You are going to lift a weight you can normally hit for each of the prescribed exercises for 6-10 reps. When you hit failure, rest for 20 seconds, repeat this again to failure, rest 20 seconds and repeat this again. This is a traditional rest-pause set, three sets in one.

Now, here is the kicker.

Immediately reduce the weight by 20-30 percent and repeat the exact same sequence. You have gone heavy and accomplished six sets in minimal time, and you will grow!

Do this for all four exercises.

A practical example for the dumbbell bench press would be:

80s x 8 reps

Rest 20 Seconds

80s x 3 reps

Rest 20 seconds

80s x 2 reps

Rest 20 seconds

60s x 7 reps

Rest 20 Seconds
60s x 4 Reps
Rest 20 Seconds
60s x 4 Reps

			Rest Pause Drop
Exercise	**Sets**	**Reps**	**Comments**
DB Bench Press	1	RPD	*Get a good stretch at the bottom to reap the benefits of this movement.*
Dips	1	RPD	*If you are unable to add weight to your bodyweight do these band assisted as a first choice, if no bands use a dip assistance machine.*
Incline Cable Fly	1	RPD	*Emphasize Stretch at the bottom; hold the top contracted position for ½ a second.*
Overhead Rope Tricep Extension	1	RPD	*Emphasize Stretch at the bottom; hold the top contracted position for ½ a second.*

Final Thoughts

You just got more done in less time without sacrificing intensity. Give this a shot without sacrificing the perils of volume or intensity.

This is not for the faint of heart.

Time to hit the pig iron!

◼ ◼ ◼
Time Under Tension — Jailhouse Strong Style

Anybody that has spent a little time in the Jailhouse and has come out Jailhouse Strong knows that when it comes to strength training, options are limited but creativity is abundant!

I am going to share a technique I learned in high school from a very big, muscular man who got big in the big house. Since then, I have successfully used it with the likes of Johnnie Jackson, Branch Warren and the corporate warriors who are low on time but high on maximizing muscularity.

Those that lack testicular fortitude, stop reading now! This is not for the faint of heart — these workouts are brutal, but also brutally effective at building muscle.

Academia's Take

Scientists, for some time, have hypothesized that muscle hypertrophy is not purely a function of rep ranges but the actual duration of the set.

One recent study from McMaster University in Canada published in the *Journal of Physiology* concluded prolonged muscle contraction was the most important variable for increasing muscle size. The study compared light loads using a tempo of one second up and one second down or using slow reps of six seconds up and six seconds down. The study concluded the slow reps were superior because of the prolonged time the muscle was under tension.

Turning to armchair academics for serious muscle-building advice must be done with a grain of salt. Science needs to be the guiding light for training. However, studies can have flaws, typically because they are performed on malnourished, sleep deprived, hard-partying college kids, and not the old heads that have been slanging serious pig iron in the trenches for years.

The aforementioned study compared explosive repetitions and slow repetitions with 30 percent of the subject's one-rep max. No one serious about getting stronger or packing on as much muscle as possible is doing 30 percent of their one-rep max for serious work sets. To put it in perspective, that would mean if you bench-press 200 pounds, you would workout with 60 pounds with a goal of packing on serious muscle.

Influencing Muscle Growth

Let's look at the training factors that influence muscle growth:

*   Mechanical Tension is related to exercise intensity (the amount of weight you are lifting). In other words, to get big you have to train heavy. Eight-time Mr. Olympia Lee Haney once said, *"The key to building massive, powerful muscles is to doggedly increase the training weights you use."* Science backs Haney, as does anecdotal evidence. I am not going to argue with Mr. Haney, and neither should you.

- Muscle damage is associated with muscle soreness; this inflammatory response aids in the muscle-building process, of course, assuming the lifter recovers properly.
- Metabolic Stress is a result of the byproducts of anaerobic metabolism in the 30-60 second range of set duration (i.e., hydrogen ions, lactate, and inorganic phosphates). In other words, lifting all-out for this duration of time, scientists believe, causes a huge spike in the anabolic hormones — growth hormone and IGF-1. Adding icing to the cake, metabolic stress increases excess post-exercise oxygen consumption, or EPOC, in other words you burn more calories at rest —expediting fat loss.

The previously mentioned study isn't a total farce.

However, it only sheds light on metabolic stress. Let's look at how we can maximize time under tension training, keeping in mind mechanical tension, muscle damage and metabolic stress.

Time Under Tension (TUT)

Time under tension training is simply performing the maxium amount of reps in the specicified time, with maximum intensity. Step on the gas! Lightweights need not apply, this is a sprint not a marathon.

Follow the below guidelines for TUT:

- Control the negative reps and explode on positives.
- The goal is to keep the weight moving, if you reach momentary muscular failure (MMF), continue with partials. DO NOT DECREASE THE WEIGHT!!
- Start with weights you can do for a true rep max of 7-11 reps, shoot for 10-15 including partial contractions.
- On each set, reduce load by approximately 1/3; so, if you start with 90 pounds, set two would be with 60 pounds and set three with 40 pounds.
- This technique is very high-intensity; do it for a maximum of three to four weeks before taking a light week.
- Weekly progression can be varied by adding 5-10 seconds per set, keeping the rest interval the same or keeping the time constant but increasing weight.
- Use primarily bilateral movements (ones that use two limbs); dumbbell movements would be with both limbs contracting simateounsly. There are exceptions to this rule. You will see two effective unilateral movements below.

The Routine

Here is a three-day-a-week time under tension routine designed for someone with minimal time who is willing to put out maximal effort for training. These routines only work if you put forth an all-out effort.

Routine Guidelines

- Superset exercises are performed consecutively
- Each exercise is maximum repetitions for 30 seconds
- Take a two-minute break after each superset
- If this isn't tough, you aren't giving 100 percent

Chest and Back TUT Workout		
Superset 1	DB Incline Press	Neutral Grip Pull Ups
Superset 2	Dips	T-Bar Chest Supported Rows
Superset 3	Chain Fly	One Armed DB Rows

Leg and Bicep TUT Workout		
Superset 1	Leg Press	Incline DB Bicep Curl
Superset 2	Leg Curl	Leg Extension
Superset 3	Bodyweight Squats	Reverse Curls

Shoulder and Tricep TUT Workout		
Superset 1	DB Military Press	DB Reverse Fly
Superset 2	DB Incline Lateral Raises	Bodyweight Skullcrushers
Superset 3	Front Raise - Plate	Lying DB Tricep Extension

Final Thoughts

Keep in mind that muscle hypertrophy is a product of muscle damage, mechanical tension and metabolic stress. The time under tension method, done with maximum intensity, exploits all three hypertrophic mechanisms. Remember, keep on moving; 1/8 of an inch is moving.

Time under tension is one more weapon at your disposal in the muscle-building war.

Time to hit the pig iron!

8 x 8 Chest Training

Bodybuilding guru turned trainer to the stars Vince Gironda boasted a clientele ranging from bodybuilding iconoclast Larry Scott to tinsel town demigod Denzel Washington.

Bodybuilding historians credit Vince with the discovery of a plethora of unique exercises still practiced by physique artists in the trenches today. These include "drag" curls, sternum chin-ups (touching the chest to the bar), bench presses to the neck, sissy squats, and dips emphasizing a forward lean.

Long before the lab confirmed the efficacy of high-volume training for hypertrophy or the emergence of any popular "new systems," Gironda aggressively expounded the gospel of high-volume training.

Gironda certainly believed that the only place success comes before work is in the dictionary. His famous high volume workouts are not three-hour marathon sessions with built-in breaks for socializing; they are fast paced, testing cardiovascular conditioning and testicular fortitude.

Vince devised a surplus of famous training routines, but his "baby" was the 8 sets of 8 reps regimen. Quoting Vince directly, *"I have a definite preference for the 8 X 8 system of sets and reps… I come back to this high intensity 'honest workout' more often than any other for maximizing muscle fiber growth in the quickest possible time for the advanced bodybuilder."*

Keep in mind, much of Vince's success was before anabolic steroids and other muscle-building drugs arrived on the scene.

To this day, there is a legion of bodybuilders that believe Gironda's 8 x8 system is second to none for concurrently adding muscle mass and shedding body fat. Gironda vehemently warns his system is not for beginners, saying, *"You have to build up to the stage where you can benefit from this extremely advanced form of training. I doubt if anyone with less than two years of training experience could benefit from this method."*

If you push as much weight as possible and stay on the prescribed rest intervals, plain and simple, this is interval training on steroids.

How it Works

This is a sprint, not a marathon!

Goals revolving around strength will not benefit from the regular use of this routine. It is for aesthetic enhancement by rapidly adding slabs of muscular beef to your frame.

You will select four exercises, with 60-65 percent of your one-repetition max (if you are good at reps, go with 65 percent, if you are poor, go with 60 percent).

You will perform this routine for four weeks; week one, you will rest 60 seconds between sets, week two you will rest 45 seconds between sets, week three you rest 35 sounds between sets and on the final week attempt 20 seconds between sets. Do not go over 30, come hell or high water.

Week one should take approximately an hour; each subsequent workout will be shorter. Stick with the same four exercises, all four weeks.

8x8 Chest Routine			
Exercise	Sets	Reps	Comments
Dips	8	8	*Lean forward and keep elbows out during the dip to put the brunt of the load on the chest. Follow outlined rest intervals weekly.*
Reverse Grip Bench Press	8	8	*This exercise is to emphasize upper chest development, a barbell or dumbbell is okay. Follow outlined rest intervals weekly.*
Flat Cable Fly	8	8	*Make sure to emphasize a full range of motion. Follow outlined rest intervals weekly.*
DB Pullover	8	8	*The dumbbell variation of the pullover shifts a majority of the load to the chest. Keep a 10-15 degree bend in the elbow throughout the entirety of the movement. Follow outlined rest intervals weekly.*

Final Thoughts

We would not recommend training this way year-round because you are not lifting heavy enough to maximize hypertrophy.

If you are stale on a conventional routine, four weeks of this type of training can interject the needed "muscle confusion" to ignite the hypertrophic switch.

Vince was an outside-the-box thinker, and he ran his gym like Attila The Hun. If he saw a member performing an exercise or using a training method he disapproved of, it was grounds for immediate dismissal from the gym.

Sometimes an unconventional strategy is needed to plow through a conventional plateau.

Time to hit the pig iron!

High-Volume Arm Blast

"The last three or four reps is what makes the muscle grow. This area of pain divides the champion from someone else who is not a champion. That's what most people lack, having the guts to go on and just say they'll go through the pain no matter what happens."
- Arnold Schwarzenegger.

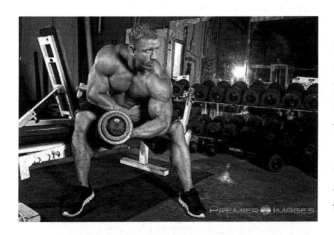

If you are the type of person that thrives on those last three or four reps that cause temporary pain and spark long-term growth, this is the workout for you. If you prefer a safer, more comfortable route, no hard feelings but I wouldn't waste your time reading the rest of the workout.

This is an old-school, high-volume arm blast! Keyboard pundits can debate between volume and intensity and what sparks growth — we will leave no stone unturned and cover both bases.

High Volume Arm Blast			
Exercise	**Sets**	**Reps**	**Comments**
Dips-Chin Ups	5	3	*Dips and chin-ups are done in a superset fashion. Go as heavy as possible on both exercises, adding weight if applicable; rest two minutes between supersets.*
Barbell Bicep Curls	6	??	*Start with 50% of your best set of eight reps, if you can do 90 pounds for eight reps, this would be 45 pounds (90 * .5=45). If your starting weight is under 60 pounds, add five pounds per set, if it is over 60 pounds add 10 pounds per set. Perform six reps at your starting weight then add the prescribed weight (five or 10 pounds) as fast as possible; do another six reps, keeping this sequence for as many sets as possible. Once you reach failure, go the opposite way by subtracting (five or 10 pounds per set).*
Skull Crushers	6	??	*See above description*
Hammer Curls	6	??	*See above description*
Overhead Rope Extension	6	??	*See above description*

Final Thoughts

This workout requires you to give a maximum effort to receive maximum benefits. Only you know when you truly cannot push on.

This workout generally should be performed once a week. Someone looking to specialize in arms or bring up a weak point can consider performing it two to three days a week.

If your arms haven't grown since WHAM! topped the pop charts, give it a shot!

Time to hit the pig iron!

■ ■ ■
Triple-Threat Arm Assault

In today's ultra-competitive IFBB pro bodybuilding circuit, 21-inch arms are considered massive. Let's go back 60 years and take a look at the first bodybuilder to build 21-inch guns, Leroy Colbert.

Leroy was born in 1933 and before he could legally drink, in 1952 at 19 years old, he was already Mr. New York. A bigger stage was out there and it had Leroy's name in bright lights; by 1953, Colbert was Mr. Eastern America.

In 1955, as things really began to get going, Leroy's competitive bodybuilding career was ended by a severe motorcycle accident.

Colbert may not have had some of the titles of other famous bodybuilders of his era, but he always had a cult-like following because of his massive arms and uncanny upper body development.

Leroy's massive arms were built before the arrival of anabolic steroids!

Sure, genetics played a role, but with such massive development, it would be naïve to not investigate and experiment with someone's methods that arguably built the greatest set of arms in the history of weight training.

Leroy trained his arms three times weekly, and each workout was 8-10 sets of biceps and 8-10 sets of triceps; he performed two exercises each for biceps and triceps. Flying in the face of most modern day science, Leroy most certainly did not look to the lab for hard data; instead, he relied on intuition and hard work.

High Volume Arm Blast			
Day 1			
Exercise	**Sets**	**Reps**	**Comments**
Bicep Curl "21's"	4	21	*Using a barbell, perform seven reps from the bottom position (arms extended) up to halfway of full flexion; next perform seven reps from halfway to full flexion, and finally perform seven full range of motion repetitions. Rest two minutes between sets.*
Weighted Dips	4	5,8,10,12	*Keep your torso upright to place emphasis on triceps; add as much additional weight as possible for each set. Rest three minutes between sets.*
DB Concentration Curl	4	6,8,10,12	*Go as heavy as possible but use 100 percent strict repetitions. Rest 90 seconds between sets.*
Overhead French Press	4	15,10,8,7	*Perform standing, Using an EZ curl bar, emphasize the stretch at the bottom of the movement. Rest 90 seconds between sets*
Day 2			
Exercise	**Sets**	**Reps**	**Comments**
Reverse Curls	4	8	*Use a barbell, go as heavy as possible, each set with strict repetitions. Rest two minutes between sets.*
Skullcrusher	4	8	*Use an EZ curl bar, lightly tap the forehead each rep, keep the elbows in tight. Go as heavy as possible but there is absolutely no room for cheating! Rest two minutes between sets*
Incline DB Curls	4	12	*Keep palms supinated through the entirety of each repetition, emphasize the stretch at the bottom of the movement holding it for half of a second. STRICT, STRICT, STRICT and go as heavy as possible without sacrificing technique or range of motion. Rest two minutes between sets.*
Bent Arm Pullovers	4	15	*Use a barbell. Emphasize the stretch, this will hammer the long head of the triceps; purposefully focus on the triceps while performing the pull over. Rest threee minutes between sets.*
Day 3			
Repeat Day 1			

Final Thoughts

If your measurements haven't improved since Bubba was getting frisky in the Oval Office, then why not give this arm blast a shot?

Sure, it may be outside your comfort zone, but how many natural pros today can match the arm development of Leroy Colbert?

Time to hit the pig iron!

The Ahrens Press

The late Perry Reader, considered one of the most notable and honest iron game historians of all-time, repeatedly noted in the 1950s and 60s that Chuck Ahrens had the widest shoulders of any human being on the face of the earth.

A cursory Google search of Chuck Ahrens reveals that Ahrens was huge, with nearly a 60-inch chest and shoulders that eclipsed the two-foot mark by four inches! Ahrens was also somewhat of a mystery man, commonly referred to as the reclusive powerhouse, lionizing his place as one of the founding fathers that put Muscle Beach on the map.

Besides extremely heavy lateral raises and overhead barbell presses, there may have been another exercise that aided in Ahrens' uncanny deltoid development.

This exercise is affectionately known as the "Ahrens Press."

The Ahrens press is a variation of the overhead dumbbell press, but instead of pressing the dumbbells straight up, you press them up and away laterally, sort of like making a V with both arms.

Necessity was the mother of invention, in this case!

Ahrens had no choice but to press the dumbbells in this style because he used special loadable dumbbells that were very long; in other words, it was impossible to press them straight because they would hit each other with the massive poundages he routinely threw overhead.

What's this mean for the modern-day bodybuilder?

Because of the lateral pressing motion, this exercise forces the medial delts or "caps" to work harder.

Exercise Description

- Grasp two dumbbells and lift them to shoulder level with a pronated grip
- From shoulder position, press the dumbbells out laterally (away from you)
- Finish with arms locked and at a 15- to 30-degree angle
- Return to starting position

					Ahrens Press
Exercise	**Sets**	**Reps**	**Intensity**	**Rest Interval**	**Comments**
Overhead Press Standing	3	3	3RM	180 Sec.	*As heavy as possible each set.*
Ahrens Press (Cluster Set)	??	5	15RM of Overhead DB Press	30 Sec.	*Start with 15 rep max of a traditional dumbbell press, do as many sets of 5 as possible with Ahrens Press.*
Incline Lateral Raise	8	8	15 RM	30 Sec.	*Emphasize stretch of the movement, no cheating whatsoever*
Reverse Pec Deck	3	3	12RM	90 Sec.	*Hold the contracted position for one second.*
Hand Stand Push Ups	3	MAX	3RM	60 Sec.	*If you are unable to do these, do them in the downward dog yoga position.*

Final Thoughts

The key to maximize muscular development is synergistically blending the most effective methods of the past with the newest innovation.

Give this oldie but goody a shot!

Time to hit the pig iron!

Blast Through Plateaus With Isometrics

For a quick review, there are three basic types of muscular contractions; concentric, eccentric, and isometric. The first two are utilized daily by lifters seeking bigger, stronger muscles. The third kind, isometric, is kind of like the redheaded step child you leave locked in the attic when you have friends over.

Three Types of Contractions

Concentric contraction is a muscular contraction occurring in conjunction with a shortening of the muscle. The bicep is concentrically contracted during the up-phase of a bicep curl.

The eccentric contraction is defined as a muscular contraction with a simultaneous lengthening of the muscle. This can be seen when lowering the dumbbell during a bicep curl.

The third type of contraction, isometric, is a muscular contraction with the muscle in a static position, no lengthening or shortening. An example of this would be your quads contracting during a wall sit.

While concentric and eccentric contractions should be your bread and butter and account for most of your workload, adding in some isometric exercises can help you break through those pesky sticking points and reach your lifting goals.

Benefits of Adding Isometrics

The biggest benefit of including isometric contractions in your training is that the amount of activation (muscle fiber recruitment) during an isometric hold is greater than both eccentric and concentric. A 2001 study by Nicholas Babault et al. found that, "The mean activation levels during maximal eccentric and maximal concentric contractions were 88.3 and 89.7%, respectively, and were significantly lower ($P < 0.05$) with respect to maximal isometric contractions (95.2%)."[3]

Isometric contractions allow the lifter to push maximally for a greater amount of time at a specified point in the lift. For example, a complete bench press will maybe take two seconds... tops. But with isometric training you can push the bar up into the pins in any position you want and contract maximally in that particular position/angle for 5-10 seconds.

This not only gets you stronger at the position you did your isometric contractions, but also at surrounding angles. A study performed by Kitai and Sale found that although strength gains were greatest at the angle where the exercise transpired, they were also seen at angles close to the one worked isometrically (+/-5 degrees).[4] So, basically, isometric contractions can help you get through sticking points, but they also get you stronger at angles before and after your sticking point.

---

[3] Babault, N., Pousson, M., Ballay, Y., & Van Hoecke, J. (2001). Activation of Human Quadriceps Femoris During Isometric, Concentric, and Eccentric Contractions. J Appl Physiol, 91, 2628-2634.

[4] Kitai, T.A., & Sale, D.G. (1989). Specificity of Joint Angle in Isometric Training. Eur J Appl Physiol, 58, 744-748

Another great benefit of isometric training is that is allows you to recruit fibers without all the wear and tear on your joints. You can work your sticking points without going through the entire range of motion; this can save your shoulders and elbows from some stress.

How to Implement Isometrics

Let's look at the bench press as an example. All of us have a sticking point in the bench press. This usually occurs about mid-range, after the explosion off the chest and before the lockout of the triceps. So, to work on this sticking point, we do our normal bench press routine, and once that is finished we add in some isometric contractions at the sticking point (this is called Maximal Effort Isometrics).

You can do this by heading over to the squat rack and putting the safety pins at the sticking point level and pushing the bar up as hard as you can against the pins. Make sure the squat rack is bolted down (or you have a fat guy with you who can sit on the rack so it won't move)!

Another interesting way to utilize isometrics is called Static-Dynamic Isometric Training. This is characterized by doing a three- to six-second isometric hold followed immediately by a dynamic full range of motion set. Static-Dynamic Isometrics have been proven to be more effective than doing only dynamic effort lifts.[5]

Isometrics should never be your meat and potatoes for the training day. They should be used as an assistance exercise two to three times per week. They are very taxing on the central nervous system and should be utilized accordingly.

4 Week Isometric Bench Blasting Routine					
		Weeks 1-4			
Day	Exercise	Sets/Reps	Sets/Reps	Sets/Reps	Sets/Reps
		Week 1	Week 2	Week 3	Week 4
Day 1	Bench Press	4x3 @ 85%	3x3 @ 87%	2x3 @ 90%	1x3 @ 92%
	Max Isometric Push at Sticking Point for 6 Seconds Followed by Speed Bench	4x3 @ 70%	6x3 @ 70%	8x3 @ 70%	10x3 @ 70%
	Wide Grip Pause Bench	3x6	3x5	3x4	3x3
	Military Press	3x6	3x6	3x6	3x6
	Incline DB Press	3x10	3x10	3x10	3x10
	Wide Fly	3x12	3x12	3x12	3x12
Day 2	Close Grip Bench	3x5	3x5	3x5	3x5
	Max Isometric Push at Sticking Point	12x8 Sec. (3 different positions x 4 reps)	12x8 Sec. (3 different positions x 4 reps)	12x8 Sec. (3 different positions x 4 reps)	12x8 Sec. (3 different positions x 4 reps)
	Dicks Press	3x8	3x8	3x8	3x8
	Skullcrushers	3x10	3x10	3x10	3x10
	Weighted Dips	3x MAX	3x MAX (Add 10 lbs from Week 1)	3x MAX (Add 10 lbs from Week 2)	3x MAX (Add 10 lbs from Week 3)

Time to hit the pig iron!

---

[5] Verkhoshanky Y.V. (1986). Fundamentals of Special Strength-Training in Sports. Sportivny Press, Livonia MI. (Original work 1977, Moscow Russia: Fizkultura I Spovt).

Supersize Your Bench with Supramaximal Eccentric Training

Supramaximal Eccentric Training (SET) is a simple idea with a long name. Basically, it is using more weight on the eccentric portion of a lift (the lowering of the bar in the bench press) than you can handle concentrically (the pressing motion in the bench press). Even more basically, it means doing heavy negatives.

The Science

Studies have shown that we can handle 20-60 percent greater loads eccentrically than we can concentrically. During traditional lifting we choose our load based on what we can complete a full lift with, and because of this the eccentric portion of our lifts are repetitively underloaded.[6]

A study by Cooke, et al. revealed greater improvements in strength after a period of maximal eccentric loading (with spotters helping on the concentric portion) versus a period of traditional. The increase in strength was accredited to larger total forces experienced by the neuromuscular system.[1]

The research shows what serious powerlifters have known for years… heavy negatives get you stronger!

Now that we have the science out of the way, let's get down to the nitty-gritty and figure out what this means to the iron warrior.

How to Incorporate SET into your Training

During SET, all we care about is that the eccentric portion of the lift and weights will far exceed your one-rep max, so spotters will be needed to help with the concentric part of the lift.

There are a couple of ways to achieve this supramaximal eccentric load.

1. The first requires at least one spotter. Load the bar with 105-115percent of your one-rep max and lower it as slowly as you can; once you lower it to your chest, have your spotter lift the weight off your chest back up to lockout.

2. The second viable way to achieve this load requires the use of weight hooks. Load the bar with less than your one-rep max (maybe about 80 percent) and then load up the weighted hooks so that the resulting sum of all the weight is 105-115 percent of your one-rep max. Set up the hooks so that they release right at the level when the bar is at your chest. Lower the bar as slowly as possible, and once at your chest the hooks with the added weight will release and you can press the bar up (or have your spotter help with the concentric portion).

Both methods achieve the same goal, but if you have a pencil-neck for a training partner, it may be safer to use the second because they will not have to lift as much weight off of you.

---

[6] Tobin, D. (2014) Advanced Strength and Power Training for the Elite Athlete. Strength and Conditioning Journal, 36, 59-65

Aside from all the physical benefits of doing heavy eccentrics, they also have a positive effect on the mental aspect of your lifting. If you have been handling 115 percent eccentrically, you will be more confident heading into your next max-out day. You know you can lower the weight under control... so now you won't be scared of it crashing down on you when you go to do a full lift!

Because of the extremely high loads involved in SET, it is not something that should be tried with the novice lifter. Make sure your base is strong so that your muscles, tendons, and ligaments are prepared to successfully handle extreme loads.

Also, heavy eccentric movements have been shown to increase DOMS and can take anywhere from 7-10 days to fully recover from. So, they should be used wisely and not more than once a week for four weeks in a row. Using SET too much can easily lead to a state of overtraining. [7]

Do a four-week cycle incorporating heavy eccentrics once a week (after your working sets of bench press), then stay away from them for six to eight weeks. Start out by using 105 percent for three sets of three to five reps.

4 Week Eccentric Based Bench Routine					
Weeks 1-4					
Day	Exercise	Sets/Reps	Sets/Reps	Sets/Reps	Sets/Reps
		Week 1	Week 2	Week 3	Week 4/Deload
Day 1	Bench Press	4x3 @ 85%	3x3 @ 87%	2x3 @ 90%	1x3 @ 92%
	Supramaximal Eccentric. Lower Weight as Slow as Possible and Get Spotter to Lift Bar Up.	3x3 @ 105%	3x2 @ 110%	5x1 @ 115%	OFF
	Incline Press	3x6	3x6	3x6	2x8 @ 60%
	Seated DB Military Press	3x10	3x10	3x10	2x10 @ 60%
	Decline DB Press	3x10	3x10	3x10	2x10 @ 60%
	Wide Fly	3x15	3x15	3x15	2x15 @ 60%

Time to hit the pig iron!

---

[7] Divakara K.(2014) Postexercise Muscle Soreness. Retrieved from: http://emedicine.medscape.com/article/313267-overview

STRONGMAN

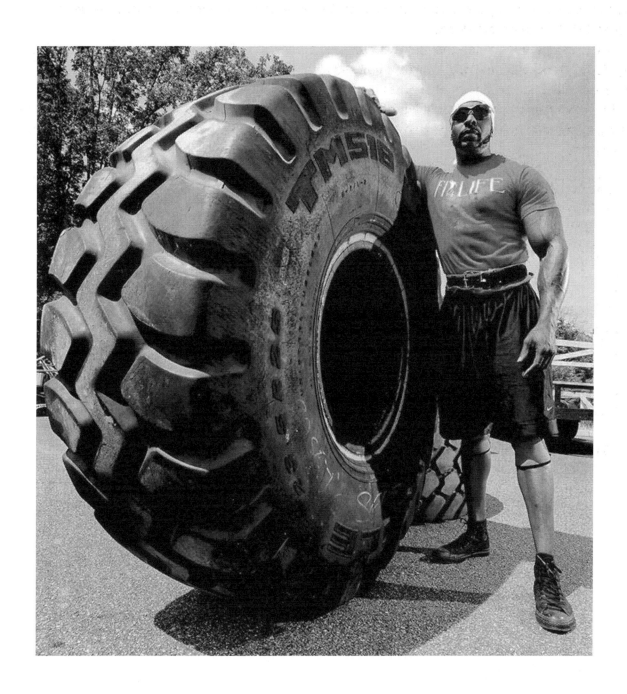

Flippin' Tractor Tires

Ever wonder why most of the newest "space age" machines at your chrome palace gym require you to sit or lay down?

Plain and simple, comfort and ease take precedence over results. Opting for the path of least resistance, though, is committing to a path of the least results.

This is a total antithesis to the tire flip.

Properly applied, the tire flip can aid in building limit strength, explosive power, slabs of muscle, flexibility and endurance to boot.

Free Equipment

Unlike purchasing the latest trendy machine that requires taking out a second mortgage and parting with your kid's college fund, tires are totally free. Any junkyard or tire yard that has tractor tires has to dispose of them and pay to do so, so you are considered a blessing to take what they consider a liability off their hands. Their liability can be one of your biggest assets in building a stronger, more powerful you.

Famous personal trainers, equipment manufacturers and chain gyms often do not mention tire flips because of the price tag. Tire flips benefit no one but you, the user.

Functionality

The tire flip is a long-time staple in strongman contests and has a huge carryover to any combative sport or sport that requires explosive power or strength. Football players and MMA athletes have reaped the benefit of forward-thinking strength coaches for years with tire flips.

Triple-extension movements are considered "functional" movements by strength coaches. Triple extension means extension of the ankles, knees, and hips — think of a vertical jump, a big hit in football or even sprinting. For decades, the go-to triple extension by the establishment is the power clean.

Tire flips force athletes into triple extension and are technically much simpler to learn than an Olympic lifting variation.

However, unlike a power clean in which you reach triple extension and then must catch the bar in a passive position on your heels, after triple extension in the tire flip, you violently push the tire down as if it were an opponent.

When you have some son-of-a-buck on his heels, put him in the ground! The tire teaches this.

Technique

Technique is not complicated but requires mastery to avoid injury. Follow these guidelines:

- Assume a four-point stance as if playing football, and set up with your chest pushing into the tire. Arms should be outside the legs, butt down and back flat.

- Like any other ground-based lift, foot position varies individual to individual; a good starting point is your most powerful vertical jump stance, for most folks this will be in the hip width range.
- From this position, lift the tire by using your hips to drive the tire upward… don't use your arms! Triple extending the ankles, knees and hips, some athletes may literally "jump."
- As you triple extend, get under the tire to catch, similar to a power clean, and from the position push the tire as fast and hard as possible away from you. Do not attempt a curl, because this where athletes have injured biceps.
- Repeat for the desired number of repetitions.
- There are variations of technique, like the sumo start (hands inside thighs) or using one knee to assist in lifting the tire as it comes up. The described technique is a great starting point; master it and then individualize it.

Starting Size

Assuming you have an understanding of technique, a good place to start and master technique is approximately your deadlift max. Remember, half the tire is ground.

Training Guidelines

Do 6-15 singles with 30-second breaks between them with a light to moderate weight for explosive power.

For strength, do sets of 1-5 reps with heavy weight. Take a full recovery between sets, and do two to four sets.

For muscle hypertrophy, do 3-5 sets of 4-8 repetitions with moderately heavy weight and rest 90-180 seconds between sets.

Final Thoughts

Tire flips can be performed as part of your legs or back workout, and if you really want to switch things up, consider an entire strongman-events day.

Build a bigger, stronger, more powerful you with tire flips.

Time to hit the pig iron!

Farmer's Walk

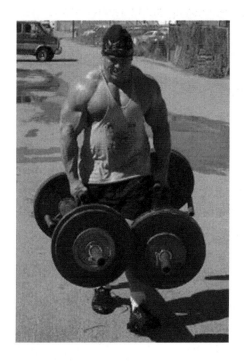

There is something special and primordially satisfying about picking up heavy implements off the ground and hauling ass.

From the alleys behind notorious German Beer Halls to the fabled "Basque Stomp", from Highland Games competitions and virtually every bush-league strongman contest to the pinnacle, World's Strongest Man, some variation of farmer's walk is used.

Functional Training

Functional training does not mean a bastardized rendition of a traditional lift with an odd object on a bosu ball — functional simply means how well a training modality transfers to the desired activity.

Anything that requires explosive power, athleticism, grip strength, overall limit strength and core strength will benefit from the farmer's walk. So, basically, the farmer's walk is the epitome of functional training for about anything.

The Exercise

The farmer's walk involves walking while holding weights at your side. As technique is mastered, the objective is no longer to walk but to move as fast as possible.

In strongman competitions and training centers, specialized farmer's walk implements are used. These can be purchased fairly inexpensively, and if you have a welder buddy he can slap a pair together with ease in no time.

No access to handles? No problem! A pair of weighted barbells or even dumbbells will work.

Go to an area with plenty of open space and set the implements parallel to one another on the floor. The handles should be approximately shoulder-width apart so you are able to stand in between them.

Reach down and grab each handle and stand back up with the implements at your side. Begin to walk forward with short, quick steps; as you are comfortable with the weight you can begin to move faster and lengthen steps. Do this for the desired distance.

Muscles Worked

Many folks classify farmer's walks as a grip test. While grip at the high level for the symmetrical, well-trained athlete will be the limiting factor, farmer's walks do, in fact, build the entire body.

Core stability, leg strength, calf strength and the strength of the entire posterior chain will be put to the test by the farmer's walk.

Implementation

If hypertrophy of the upper back and traps is the objective, use straps! Since grip is the limit factor, why limit the growth of your traps?

One outstanding trap growth strategy is supersetting barbell shrugs with farmer's walks, using straps on both exercises while going as heavy as possible. Do three to four supersets of a 75-foot farmer's walk, followed immediately by 12 barbell shrugs.

For more "functional" athleticism, ditch the straps because as your grip is challenged your forearms will grow by default. Want to really zero in on the forearms? Perform 3-4 sets of farmer's walks pinching plates, squeezing the plates together and holding the smooth part.

If strength is the primary objective, do 2-3 sets of 30-100 feet with heavy weight and full recovery between sets.

For the hypertrophic objective, do 100-200 feet for 3-4 sets (rest 90-180 seconds between sets) and use moderately heavy weight.

Final Thoughts

Farmer's walks can be part of a legs or back day. If you really want to try something wild, do an entire strongman events day.

Furthermore, farmer's walks can aid in taking your physique and functionality to a fundamentally new level.

For the bouncer at the kick-and-stab honky tonk to the lady that wants to improve her tennis game, look no further than the farmer's walk.

Time to hit the pig iron!

Conclusion

Whether your goals are performance-based, strength-based, cosmetic, improving your health, or like most folks, a combination, there is a program in this book that will help you achieve your goals.

It is important to keep a training journal and write down all of your workouts, keeping detailed notes on what is working and what is not. Learning both what works for you and, just as importantly, what doesn't work for you is key to your success.

Keep in mind everyone is unique and will react differently to the programs presented. Attack everything with an open mind and you will learn what works best for you.

Remember, there is no such thing as failure — only results!

Once again, we thank you for letting us be a part of your training journey.

Questions and feedback are always welcomed. We look forward to hearing about the success of your journey.

www.joshstrength.com
www.noahstrength.com

Photo Credits

Thank you to the following people for providing us pictures to use for this project:

Shannon Skinner, Owner of Premier Images: http://m.facebook.com/shannon.skinner2
Dave Luyando, Owner of Luyando Photography: www.daveluyando.com
Iron Rebel Power Gear: http://www.ironrebel.com/
Brian Dobson, Owner of Metroflex Gym: http://www.metroflexgym.com/
Dan Bryant
Brandi Whitehead
Orlando Green
Thank you to the following people for allowing us to use their image (s):
BJ Whitehead
TJ Clark
Max Fairchild (Cover Model)
Lou Moreira
Tyrus Hughes
Josh Bryant
Brian Dobson
Orlando Green

Printed in Great Britain
by Amazon.co.uk, Ltd.,
Marston Gate.